Mediterranean Taste

*Ideas For A Better Alimentation
Starting From Handpicked Recipes You
Will Never Forget!*

Mediterranean Flavor

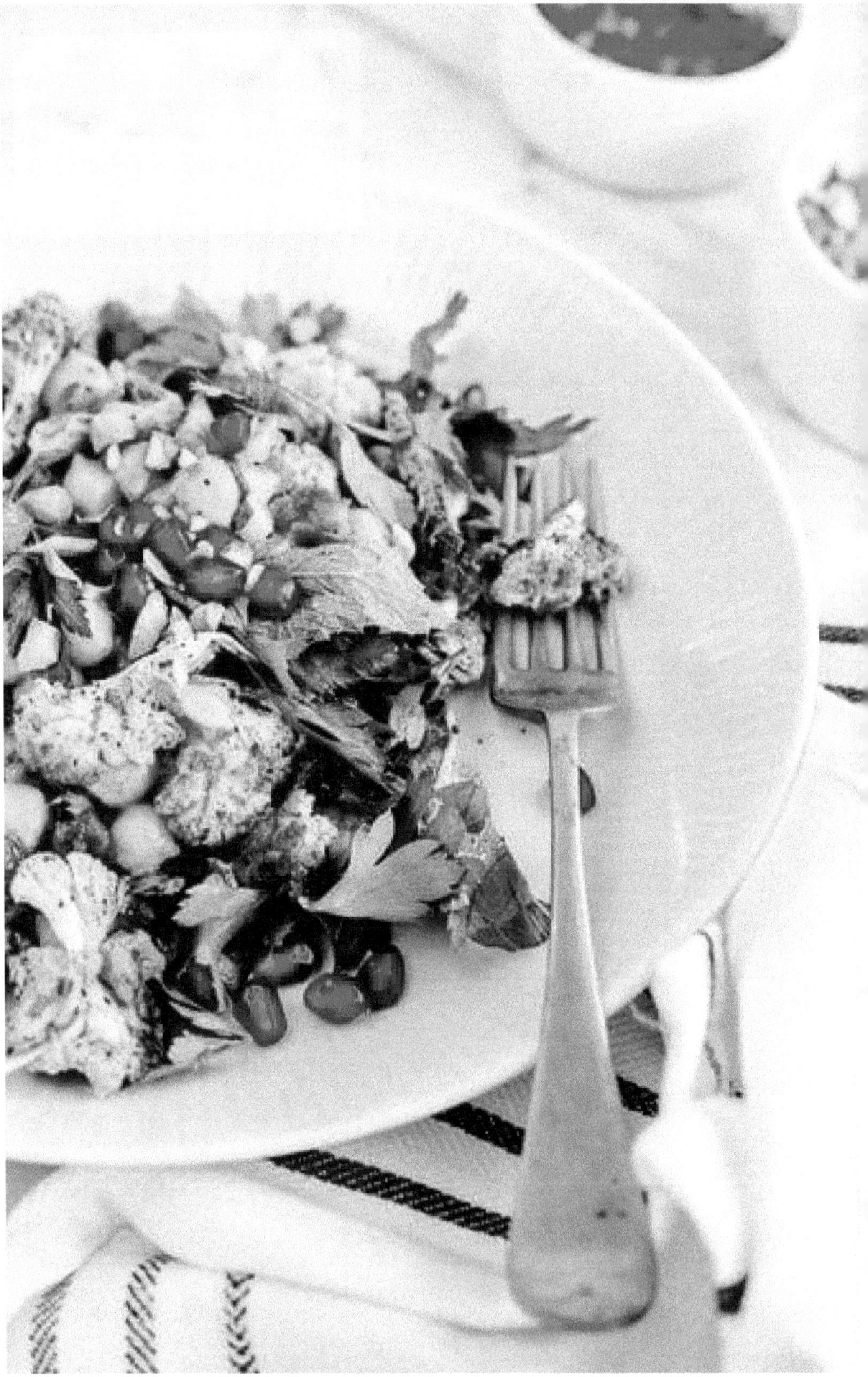

the publisher or the original author of this work can be in any fashion deemed liable for any hardship or damages that may befall them after undertaking the information described herein.

Additionally, the information in the following pages is intended only for informational purposes and should thus be thought of as universal. As befitting its nature, it is presented without assurance regarding its prolonged validity or interim quality. Trademarks that are mentioned are done without written consent and can in no way be considered an endorsement from the trademark holder.

Table of Contents

INTRODUCTION

The Mediterranean Diet is the traditional diet of the countries surrounding the Mediterranean Sea, such as Greece, Spain, and Italy. It focuses on the regional foods from those countries, which have many benefits, including improving heart health, chronic disease, and obesity.

The Mediterranean Diet reflects the personality of these regions and includes a wonderful variety of ingredients and recipes, featuring grains, fats from fish, olive oil, nuts, fruits, and lean meats. It is easy to follow and will provide lots of healthy and delicious meals that your family will love.

This diet is generally characterized by a high intake of plant-based food such as fresh fruits, vegetables, nuts and cereals, and olive oil, with a moderate amount of fish and poultry, and a small amount of dairy products, red meats, and sweets. Wine is allowed with every meal but at a moderate level. The Mediterranean Diet focuses strongly on social and cultural activities like communal mealtimes, resting after eating, and physical activities.

The Mediterranean Diet is not simply a weight loss or fad diet; however, raising your dietary fiber and cutting down on red meat, animal fats, and processed foods will lead to weight loss and a decreased risk of many diseases.

The Mediterranean Diet Pyramid

The Mediterranean Diet Pyramid is a visual tool that summarizes the diet. It suggests pattern of eating and gives guidelines for meal frequency and food management. This pyramid allows you to develop healthy eating habits and maintain calorie counts as well.

The pyramid tiers consist of the following groups:

- **Plant-based foods**

This includes olive oil, fruits, vegetables, whole grains, legumes, beans, nuts and seeds, and spices and herbs. These foods should be part of every meal. Olive oil is the main fat used in cooking. It can occasionally be replaced with butter or cooking oil, but in smaller quantities.

Fresh herbs and spices can be used in generous amounts in dishes for enhancing taste and as an alternative to salt. Dried herbs can also be used. Fresh ginger and garlic are always allowed for flavor.

- **Seafood**

Seafood is an important staple and one of the main sources of protein in the Mediterranean Diet. Make sure you have seafood at least twice a week. There are many varieties of fish that will work, as well as mussels, shrimps, and crab. Tuna is a great source of protein and works well in sandwiches and salads.

- **Dairy and Poultry**

Yogurt, milk, cheese, and poultry can be consumed at a moderate level. If you use eggs in cooking and baking, include them in your weekly limit. Choose healthy cheese options like ricotta, feta, and parmesan. You can have them as toppings and garnishing your meals and dishes.

- **Sweets and Red Meat**

Sweets and meats are used less in this diet. If you eat them, cut down on the quantity and choose lean meat. Red meat, sugar, and fat are not good for heart health and blood sugar.

- **Water**

The Mediterranean Diet encourages increased daily water intake, 9 8-ounce glasses for women and 13 for men. For pregnant and breastfeeding women, the amount should be higher.

- **Wine**

The Mediterranean Diet allows for moderate wine consumption with meals. Alcohol reduces the risk of heart disease. One glass of wine for women and two for men is the recommended daily limit.

Foods That Are Not Allowed in the Mediterranean Diet

This diet satisfies your food cravings by providing better alternatives. It helps you to shift your mindset from looking for snacks to having fresh fruits and vegetables that will satisfy your between-meal hunger.

The following items should be restricted or replaced by healthy options:

- **Added sugar**

Sugar is one of the most difficult items to avoid in your diet. Try to stick to healthy sugar from fresh fruits and vegetables. Avoid processed foods; the added sugars in pasta sauce, peanut butter, fruit juices, bread, and bakery products are considered empty calories.

Added sugars are commonly used in processed food like:

- High fructose corn syrup
- Glucose
- Corn syrup

- Sucrose
- Maltose
- Corn sweetener

You can add fresh fruits like strawberries and raspberries to your water for flavor and refreshment as well as eating them. Switch to an organic sweetener like honey or maple syrup instead of using refined sugars.

- **Refined grains**

Refined grains are prohibited in the Mediterranean Diet because they lead to heart disease and type 2 diabetes. Grains are often grouped with carbohydrates, but they do not fall into the "bad carbs" category until they are refined. Refined grains go through a milling process during which the major nutrients are removed. They are left with less fiber, iron, and vitamins and more empty calories.

The most common refined grains consist of:

- White flour
- White bread
- White rice
- White flour pizza crust

- **Breakfast cereals**

Whole grains are a better alternative. When possible, choose sourdough bread. Enjoy sandwiches in a whole-grain wrap or pita bread. You can also try plant-based alternatives like cauliflower crust, cauliflower rice, or spiralized vegetables in place of pasta. Swap in whole grains like quinoa and brown rice.

- **Refined Oils**

Refined oils are extremely damaging to your health. The key nutrients have been stripped from out and additional chemicals added in, making their way to your food.

Most oils are extracted from the seeds of plants. This includes soybean oil, corn oil, sunflower oil, peanut oil, and olive oil. Vegetable oils are a combination of multiple plants. The process of extracting the oil involves a variety of chemicals that can increase inflammation in the body. The fat that remains in the oil has been linked to several health conditions such as cancer, heart disease, and diabetes. Oils are also used to create margarine in a hydrogenation process, using chemicals that allow the oil to remain in a solid-state. When the oil is hydrogenated, the fatty acids that were in the oil are further destroyed and transformed into trans fatty acids. Several scientific studies have been conducted to show the connection of trans fatty acids to some debilitating health conditions.

Trans fatty acids are considered to be some of the unhealthiest fats you can consume, especially when it comes to your heart. These industrially manufactured fats cause LDL cholesterol to increase. High amounts of LDL or bad cholesterol can clog and destroy your arteries and increase blood pressure. This significantly increases your risk of heart attack and stroke.

Some of the most common trans fats or hydrogenated oils that you might not be aware of include:

- Microwaveable popcorn
- Butter
- Margarine
- Vegetable oil
- Fried foods
- Pre-packaged muffins, cakes, doughnuts, and pastries
- Coffee creamers
- Prepared pizza dough or pizza crust
- Cake frosting
- Potato chips
- Crackers

The Mediterranean Diet focuses on replacing these refined oils and processed foods with more wholesome and natural ingredients. Refined oils can be easy to eliminate from your diet. If you are used to sautéing your foods with refined oil, switch to unrefined olive oil. Instead of frying foods in oil, bake or grill them.

- **Processed Meat**

Processed meats have been processed extensively to preserve flavors and provide a longer shelf life. The most common forms are bacon, hot dogs, deli meats, sausage, and canned meats. Consuming processed meat daily can cause or increase the risk of colorectal cancer, stomach cancer, pancreatic cancer, and prostate cancer.

Sodium is what makes processed meats so harmful. Sodium is well known to increase blood pressure, which increases the risk of different heart diseases. Processed meat contains at least 50 percent more preservatives than unprocessed meats. These preservatives affect sugar tolerances and can cause insulin resistance, which can lead to diabetes.

- Switch out processed meats and red meats for fish or poultry.
- Use vegetables or beans in place of meat.

- Use a variety of spices to add more flavor to a dish where you would use meat in the same way.
- Spices like cumin, coriander, peppercorn, and marjoram add unique flavors to the dish so you won't miss the bacon, sausage, or ground meat.
- You can use different seasonings on sautéed or baked vegetables.
- Add roasted chickpeas or toasted seeds and nuts to dishes for more texture. These can be great alternatives to dishes that call for bacon crumbles.

Common Mistakes in the Mediterranean Diet:

When you start a new diet, you will make some mistakes or encounter situations in which you don't know what to do. Before you get on the Mediterranean Diet plan, here is a heads-up about common mistakes that people make. If you know about these mistakes, you can avoid them and achieve success more quickly.

- **All or Nothing**

Your attitude toward your diet matters a lot. This is why you must make sure you are mentally prepared for it. It will be different from your ordinary lifestyle, which is why you need an abundance of information. To learn the benefits of this diet, you can ask the experts or people who have experienced it.

- **Eating the Same Things**

Don't eat the same things over and over again, day after day. One of the most common mistakes people make is that they think that eating the same kind of vegetables all week long will help them lose weight. You must have variety in your diet. The Mediterranean Diet allows you to have multiple kinds of dishes throughout the week, but maintain portion control.

- **Deprivation**

Another mistake people make is thinking that deprivation is the only way to lose weight. The main point of this diet plan is to give you energy while helping you lose weight. Deprivation will only make you weaker. This diet plan won't work if you don't eat at all, so be sure to keep this in mind.

- **Giving up**

Don't give up in the middle of the Mediterranean Diet. If you see yourself losing weight and you think, *now I can cheat a little* ... resist. Since you've put so much effort into it already, don't give up now. If you have chocolate cravings, find a healthy alternative. It's easier to develop self-control if you can see the results, so keep your goals in mind and stay strong. Our bodies need time to adjust and stabilize in terms of the food we eat, so switching back and forth is never a good option.

- **Not setting goals**

One of the main mistakes people make is not setting goals when they start the diet. You must have a goal in terms of how much weight you want to lose and work toward it. When you don't have a plan, you will become distracted and be unable to reach your destination, no matter how hard you try.

- **Following the wrong plan**

Another common mistake is that you don't have enough knowledge about the plan you are following to lose weight. Maybe you are following the wrong plan, one that doesn't seem to work for you. If you're confused, don't decide by yourself to follow the Mediterranean Diet; consult an expert who can advise you on what to eat and do to adopt a healthy lifestyle. Many people try to keep their old habits while mixing in elements of the Mediterranean Diet, but if you don't follow the diet, you won't achieve the optimal results. Decide if you're willing to do it, and then do it right.

Your Mediterranean Shopping Guide

Apart from knowing how to start your diet, it is necessary to know a little about how to set-up your food charts.

What to have:

- Fresh vegetables: tomatoes, kale, spinach, cauliflower, Brussels sprouts, cucumbers, etc.
- Fresh fruits: An orange, apples, pears, grapes, dates, strawberries, figs, peaches, etc.
- Seeds and nuts: almonds, walnuts, cashews, sunflower seeds, etc.
- Legumes: beans, lentils, chickpeas, etc.
- Roots: yams, turnips, sweet potatoes, etc.
- Whole grains: whole oats, rye, brown rice, corn, barley, buckwheat, whole wheat, whole grain pasta, and bread
- Fish and seafood: sardines, salmon, tuna, shrimp, mackerel, oyster, crab, clams, mussels, etc.
- Poultry: turkey, chicken, duck, etc.
- Eggs—chicken, duck, quail
- Dairy products such as cheese, Greek yogurt, etc.

- Herbs and spices: mint, basil, garlic, rosemary, cinnamon, sage, pepper, etc.
- Healthy fats and oil: extra virgin olive oil, avocado oil, olives, etc.

What to avoid:

- Foods with added sugar like soda, ice cream, candy, table sugar, etc.
- Refined grains like white bread or pasta made with refined wheat
- Margarine and similar processed foods that contain trans fats
- Refined oil such as cottonseed oil, soybean oil, etc.
- Processed meat such as hot dogs, sausages, bacon, etc.
- Highly processed food with labels such as "Low-Fat" or "Diet," or anything that is not natural

Useful Information about Healthy Foods

1. Oils

The Mediterranean Diet emphasizes healthy oils. The following are some of the oils that you might want to consider.

- **Coconut oil:** Coconut oil is semi-solid at room temperature and can be used for months without turning sour. Coconut oil also has a lot of health benefits as lauric acid, which can help to improve cholesterol levels and kill various pathogens.

- **Extra-virgin olive oil:** Olive oil is well-known worldwide as one of the healthiest oils, and it is a key ingredient in the Mediterranean Diet. Olive oil can help to improve health biomarkers such as increasing HDL cholesterol and lowering the amount of bad LDL cholesterol.

- **Avocado oil:** Avocado oil is very similar to olive oil and has similar health benefits. It can be used for many purposes as an alternative to olive oil (such as in cooking).

2. Healthy salt alternatives and spices

Aside from replacing healthy oils, the Mediterranean Diet will allow you to opt for healthy salt alternatives as well.

- **Sunflower seeds**

Sunflower seeds are excellent and give a nutty and sweet flavor.

- **Fresh squeezed lemon**

Lemon is packed with Vitamin C, which helps to neutralize damaging free radicals from the system.

- **Onion powder**

Onion powder is a dehydrated ground spice made from an onion bulb, which is mostly used as a seasoning and is a fine salt alternative.

- **Black pepper**

Black pepper is also a salt alternative that is native to India. It is made by grinding whole peppercorns.

- **Cinnamon**

Cinnamon is well-known as a savory spice and available in two varieties: Ceylon and Chinese. Both of them sport a sharp, warm, and sweet flavor.

- **Fruit-infused vinegar**

Fruit-infused vinegar or flavored vinegar can give a nice flavor to meals. These are excellent ingredients to add a bit of flavor to meals without salt.

Eating Out on the Mediterranean Diet

It might seem a bit confusing, but eating out at a restaurant while on a Mediterranean Diet is pretty easy. Just follow the simple rules below:

- Try to ensure that you choose seafood or fish as the main dish of your meal
- When ordering, try to make a special request and ask the restaurant to fry their food using extra virgin olive oil
- Ask for only whole-grain based ingredients if possible
- If possible, try to read the menu before going to the restaurant
- Try to have a simple snack before you go out; this will help prevent you from overeating.

BREAKFAST

Spinach, Ham & Egg in a Mug

8 Servings

Preparation Time: 35 minutes

Ingredients

- 2 tbsps olive oil
- 2 tbsps unsalted butter, melted
- 2 pounds fresh baby spinach
- 8 eggs
- 8 tsps milk
- 14-ounce ham, sliced
- Salt and black pepper, to taste

Directions

- Preheat the air fryer to 360 degrees f and grease 8 ramekins with butter.
- Heat oil in a skillet on medium heat and add spinach.
- Cook for about 3 minutes and drain the liquid completely from the spinach.
- Divide the spinach into prepared ramekins and layer with ham slices.

- Crack 1 egg over ham slices into each ramekin and drizzle evenly with milk.
- Sprinkle with salt and black pepper and bake for about 20 minutes.

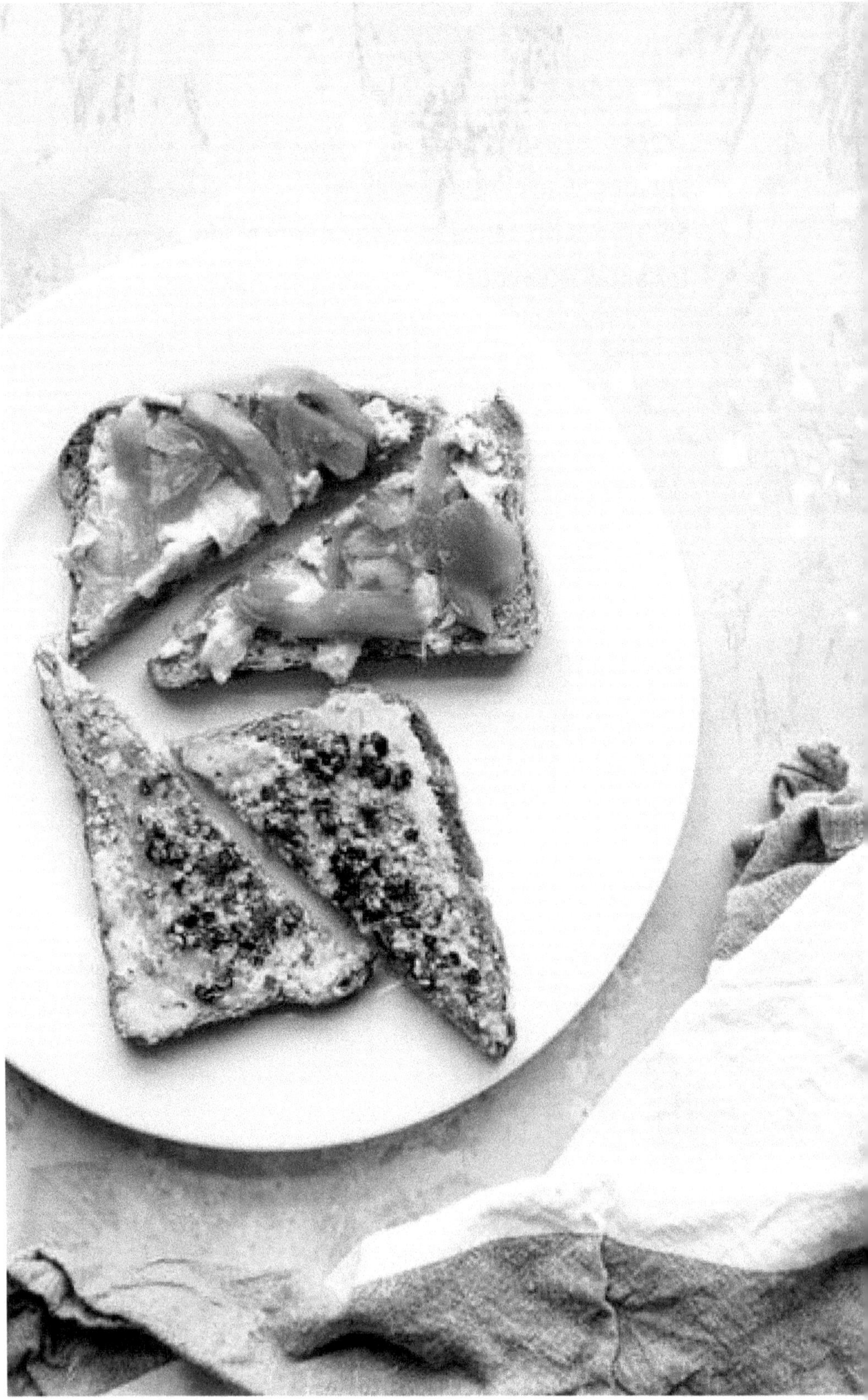

Sausage & Bacon with Eggs

2 Servings

Preparation Time: 25 minutes

Ingredients

- 4 chicken sausages
- 4 bacon slices
- 2 eggs
- Salt and freshly ground black pepper, to taste

Directions

- Preheat the air fryer to 330 degrees f and place sausages and bacon slices in an air fryer basket.
- Cook for about 10 minutes and lightly grease 2 ramekins.
- Crack 1 egg in each prepared ramekin and season with salt and black pepper.
- Cook for about 10 minutes and divide sausages and bacon slices on serving plates.

Steamy Almond Pancakes

8 Servings

Preparation Time: 15 minutes

Ingredients

- 2 cups creamy milk
- 3½ cups almond flour
- 1 tsp baking soda
- ½ tsp salt
- 1 tsp allspice
- 2 tbsps vanilla
- 1 tsp cinnamon
- 1 tsp baking powder
- ½ cup club soda

Directions

- Preheat the air fryer at 290 degrees f and grease the cooking basket of the air fryer.
- Whisk together salt, almond flour, baking soda, allspice, and cinnamon in a large bowl.
- Mix the vanilla, baking powder, and club soda and add to the flour mixture.

- Mix the mixture thoroughly and pour the mixture into the cooking basket.
- Cook for about 10 minutes and dish out on a serving platter.

Hot Dogs and Bacon Omelet

4 Servings

Preparation Time: 15 minutes

Ingredients

- Hot dogs chopped up
- 8 eggs
- 2 bacon slices chopped up
- 1 small onion chopped up

Directions

- Preheat the air fryer to 325 degrees f.
- Crack the eggs in an air fryer baking pan and beat well.
- Mix in the remaining ingredients and cook for about 10 minutes until completely done.

Toasted Crispy Bagels

6 Servings

Preparation Time: 10 minutes

Ingredients

- 6 tsps butter
- 6 Bagels cut in halves

Directions

- Preheat the air fryer to 375 degrees f and arrange the bagels into an air fryer basket.
- Cook for about 3 minutes and remove the bagels from the air fryer.
- Spread batter evenly over bagels and cook for about 3 more minutes.

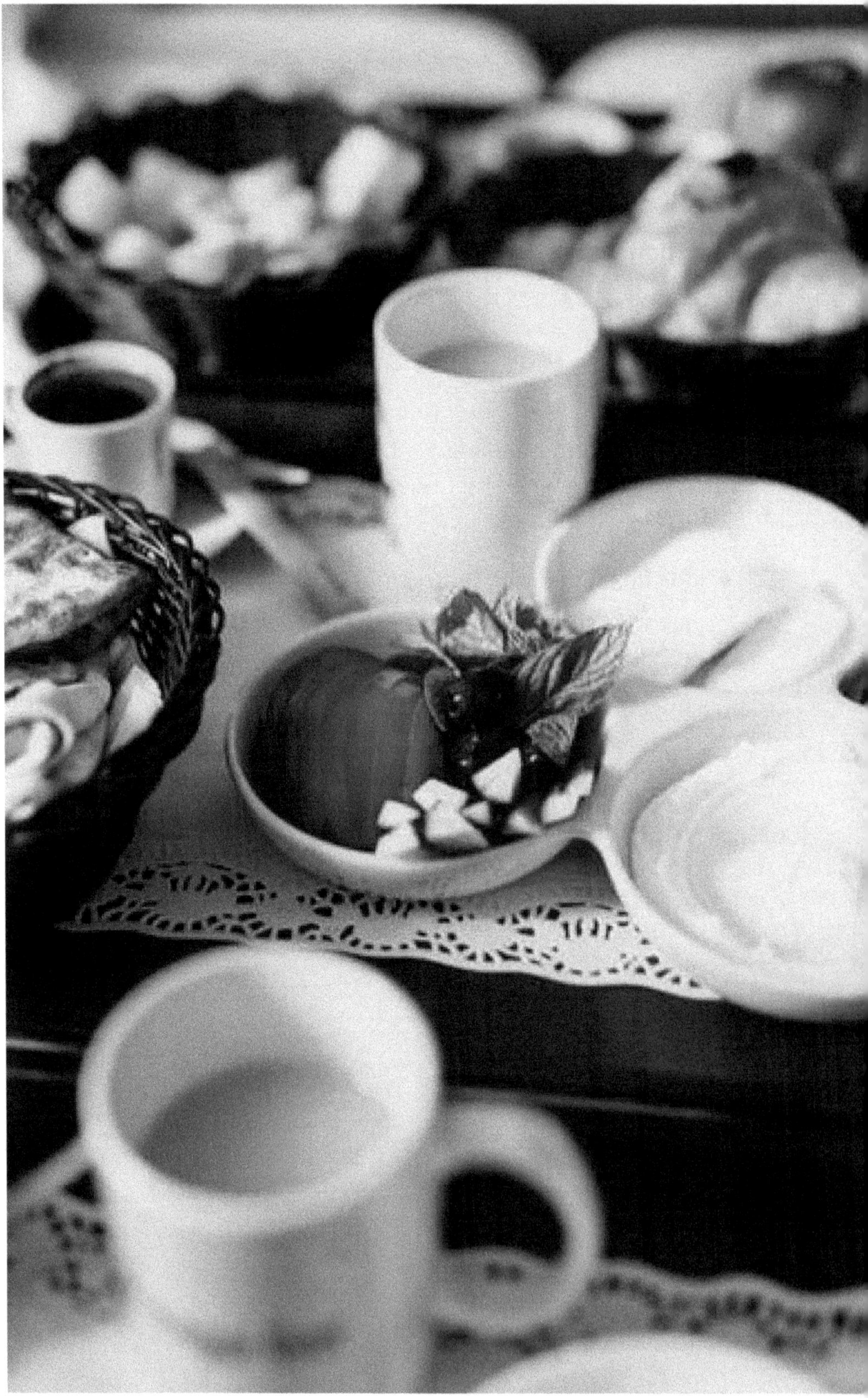

Eggless Bacon and Spinach Quiche

8 Servings

Preparation Time: 20 minutes

Ingredients

- 1 cup fresh spinach chopped up
- 8 slices of bacon cooked and chopped up
- ½ cup mozzarella cheese, shredded
- 8 tbsps milk
- Few dashes tabasco sauce
- 1 cup parmesan cheese, shredded
- Salt and freshly ground black pepper, to taste

Directions

- Preheat the air fryer to 325 degrees f and grease a baking dish.
- Put all the ingredients in a bowl and mix well.
- Pour the mixture into a prepared baking dish and cook for about 8 minutes.
- Dish out and serve.

Buttery Ham Casserole

4 Servings

Preparation Time: 25 minutes

Ingredients

- 4-ounce ham sliced finely
- 4 tsps unsalted butter, softened
- 8 large eggs, divided
- 4 tbsps heavy cream
- ¼ tsp smoked paprika
- 4 tsps fresh chives, minced
- Salt and freshly ground black pepper, to taste
- 6 tbsps parmesan cheese grated finely

Directions

- Preheat the air fryer to 325 degrees f and spread butter in the pie pan.
- Place ham slices in the bottom of the pie pan.
- Whisk together 2 eggs, cream, salt, and black pepper until smooth.
- Place the egg mixture evenly over the ham slices and crack the remaining eggs on top.
- Season with paprika, salt, and black pepper.

- Top evenly with chives and cheese and place the pie pan in an air fryer.
- Cook for about 12 minutes and serve with toasted bread slices.

Bacon and Sausage with Beans

12 Servings

Preparation Time: 30 minutes

Ingredients

- 12 medium sausages
- 12 bacon slices
- 8 eggs
- 2 cans baked beans
- 12 bread slices, toasted

Directions

- Preheat the air fryer at 325 degrees f and place sausages and bacon in a fryer basket.
- Cook for about 10 minutes and place the baked beans in a ramekin.
- Place eggs in another ramekin and the air fryer to 395 degrees f.
- Cook for about 10 more minutes and divide the sausage mixture, beans, and eggs on serving plates.
- Serve with bread slices.

French Egg Toasts

4 Servings

Preparation Time: 15 minutes

Ingredients

- ½ cup evaporated milk
- 4 eggs
- 6 tbsps sugar
- ¼ tsp vanilla extract
- 8 bread slices
- 2 tsps olive oil

Directions

- Preheat the air fryer to 395 degrees f and grease a pan.
- Put all the ingredients in a large sheet dish except the bread slices.
- Beat till well combined and dip each bread slice in egg mixture from both sides.
- Arrange the bread slices in the prepared pan and cook for about 3 minutes per side.

Colorful Veggie Hash

8 Servings

Preparation Time: 55 minutes

Ingredients

- 2 medium onions chopped up
- 2 tsps dried thyme, crushed
- 2 tsps butter
- 1 green bell pepper seeded and chopped up
- Pounds russet potatoes, peeled and chopped up
- Salt and freshly ground black pepper, to taste
- 10 eggs

Directions

- Preheat the air fryer to 395 degrees f and grease the air fryer pan with butter.
- Add bell peppers and onions and cook for about 5 minutes.
- Add the herbs, potatoes, salt, and black pepper and cook for about 30 minutes.
- Heat a greased skillet on medium heat and add beaten eggs.

- Cook for about 1 minute on each side and remove from the skillet.
- Cut it into small pieces and add egg pieces into the air fryer pan.
- Cook for about 5 more minutes and dish out.

Parmesan Garlic Rolls

4 Servings

Preparation Time: 15 minutes

Ingredients

- 1 cup parmesan cheese, grated
- 4 dinner rolls
- 4 tbsps unsalted butter, melted
- 1 tbsp garlic bread seasoning mix

Directions

- Preheat the air fryer at 360 degrees f and cut the dinner rolls into cross style.
- Stuff the slits evenly with the cheese and coat the tops of each roll with butter.
- Sprinkle with the seasoning mix and cook for about 5 minutes until cheese is fully melted.

Savory Pickled Toasts

4 Servings

Preparation Time: 25 minutes

Ingredients

- 4 tbsps unsalted butter, softened
- 8 bread slices, toasted
- 4 tbsps pickle
- ½ cup parmesan cheese, grated

Directions

- Preheat the air fryer to 385 degrees f and place the bread slice in a fryer basket.
- Cook for about 5 minutes and spread the batter evenly over bread slices.
- Layer with Branston pickle and top evenly with cheese.
- Cook for about 5 minutes until cheese is fully melted.

Eggplant and Panini Caponata

4 Servings

Preparation Time: 10 minutes

Ingredients

- ¼ cup packed fresh basil leaves.
- ¼ of a 7ounce can of eggplant caponata
- 4 ounces finely sliced mozzarella
- 1 tbsp olive oil
- 1 ciabatta roll 6-7-inch length, horizontally split

Directions

- Spread oil evenly on the sliced part of the ciabatta and layer on the following: cheese, caponata, basil leaves, and cheese again before covering with another slice of ciabatta.
- Then grill the sandwich in a panini press until cheese melts and bread gets crisped and ridged.

LUNCH

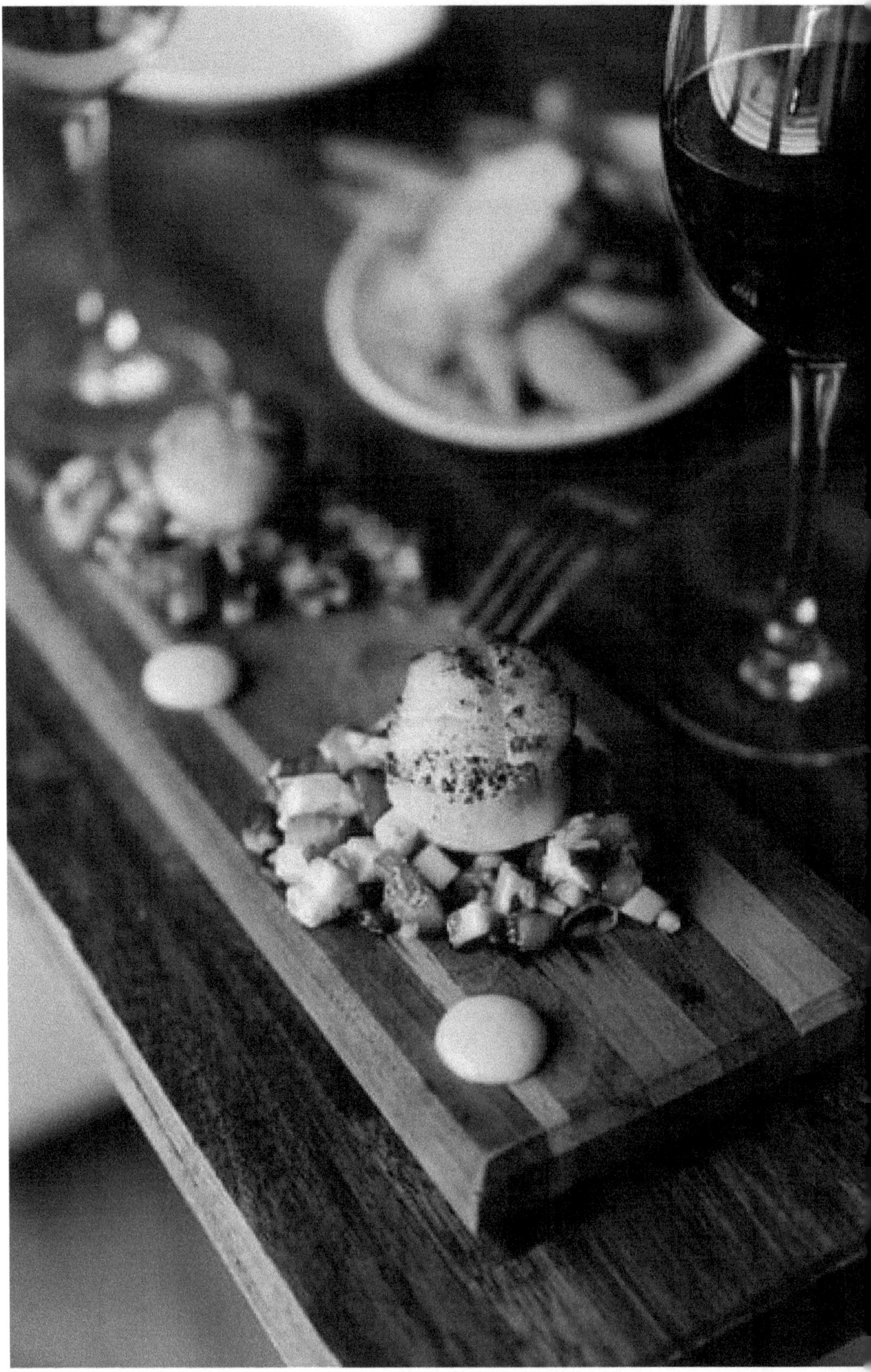

Chicken in Lettuce Wraps

6 Servings

Preparation Time: 20 minutes

Ingredients

- 5 large eggs
- 1 ½ tbsps olive oil
- 12 romaine lettuce leaves
- 1 ½ pounds chicken breasts, cubed
- 2 cups water
- 8 tbsps natural yogurt
- 3 tomatoes, seeded and chopped
- Salt and black pepper to taste

Directions

- Cover the chicken cubes with olive oil, salt, and black pepper.

- Spread evenly on a greased baking dish and place in the oven.

- Bake the chicken in the oven at 400ºF until cooked and golden brown about 8 minutes.

- Boil the eggs in salted water in a pot over medium heat for 10 minutes.

- After boiling, put the eggs in cold water, peel, and chop into small pieces. Then transfer to a bowl.

- Remove the chicken from the oven, cool it for a few minutes, and add to the eggs.

- Add the tomatoes and yogurt; mix well.

- Layer two lettuce leaves as cups and fill with two tbsps of egg mixture each.

- Serve with chilled blueberry juice.

Baked Italian Sausage with Toasted Cheese
7 Servings

Preparation Time: 20 minutes

Ingredients

- 19 oz Italian pork sausage, chopped
- 4 tbsps olive oil
- 4 green bell peppers, seeded and chopped
- 9 oz mozzarella cheese, grated
- 3 tbsps fresh parsley, chopped
- 1 ½ onions, sliced
- 5 sun-dried tomatoes, sliced thin
- 3 orange bell peppers, seeded and chopped
- A pinch of red pepper flakes
- Salt and black pepper to taste

Directions

- Heat the olive oil in a pan and cook the sausage slices for 3 minutes over medium heat, cook on each side, then remove to a bowl.

- Preheat oven to 340ºF.

- In the pan, add tomatoes, bell peppers, and onion, and cook for 5 minutes.

- Sprinkle with pepper, pepper flakes, and salt and mix well.

- Cook for 1 minute, and remove from heat.

- Spread the sausage slices into a baking dish, put the bell peppers mixture on top, scatter with the mozzarella cheese, and bakes for 10 minutes until the cheese melts.

- Sprinkle with parsley and serve.

Crispy Vegetable Frittata
6 Servings

Preparation Time: 20 minutes

Ingredients

- 12 eggs
- 3 tbsps olive oil
- 1½ carrots, chopped
- 1 cup green onion, chopped
- 1½ zucchinis, chopped
- 3 garlic cloves, minced
- 1 ½ jalapeño peppers, chopped
- 1 ½ bell peppers, seeded and chopped
- 1 tsp dried thyme
- Salt and black pepper to taste

Directions

- Heat the olive oil in a pan over medium heat.

- Add in green onions and garlic and stir for 3 minutes.

- Preheat the oven to 350ºF.

- Add in carrot, zucchini, bell pepper, and jalapeno pepper, and cook for more 4 minutes.

- Remove the mixture to a greased baking pan with cooking spray.

- In a bowl, beat the eggs, sprinkle with salt and pepper, and pour over vegetables.

- Bake for about 18 minutes.

- Serve until it's hot.

Roasted Pork with Kale Sauce

6 Servings

Preparation Time: 40 minutes

Ingredients

- 1 cup water
- 1½ pounds pork loin
- 20 oz kale, chopped
- 3 tbsps olive oil
- 3 garlic cloves, minced
- 1 tsp dry mustard
- 1½ tsps hot red pepper flakes
- 1 lemon sliced
- Salt and black pepper to taste

Directions

- Add the pork into a bowl and mix with salt, mustard, and black pepper to coat.

- Warm the oil in a saucepan over medium heat, brown the pork on all sides for 10 minutes.

- Transfer to the baking pan and roast for 1 hour at 390°F.

- In the saucepan, add kale, lemon slices, garlic, and water; cook for 10 minutes.
- Serve on a platter and sprinkle pan juices on top.

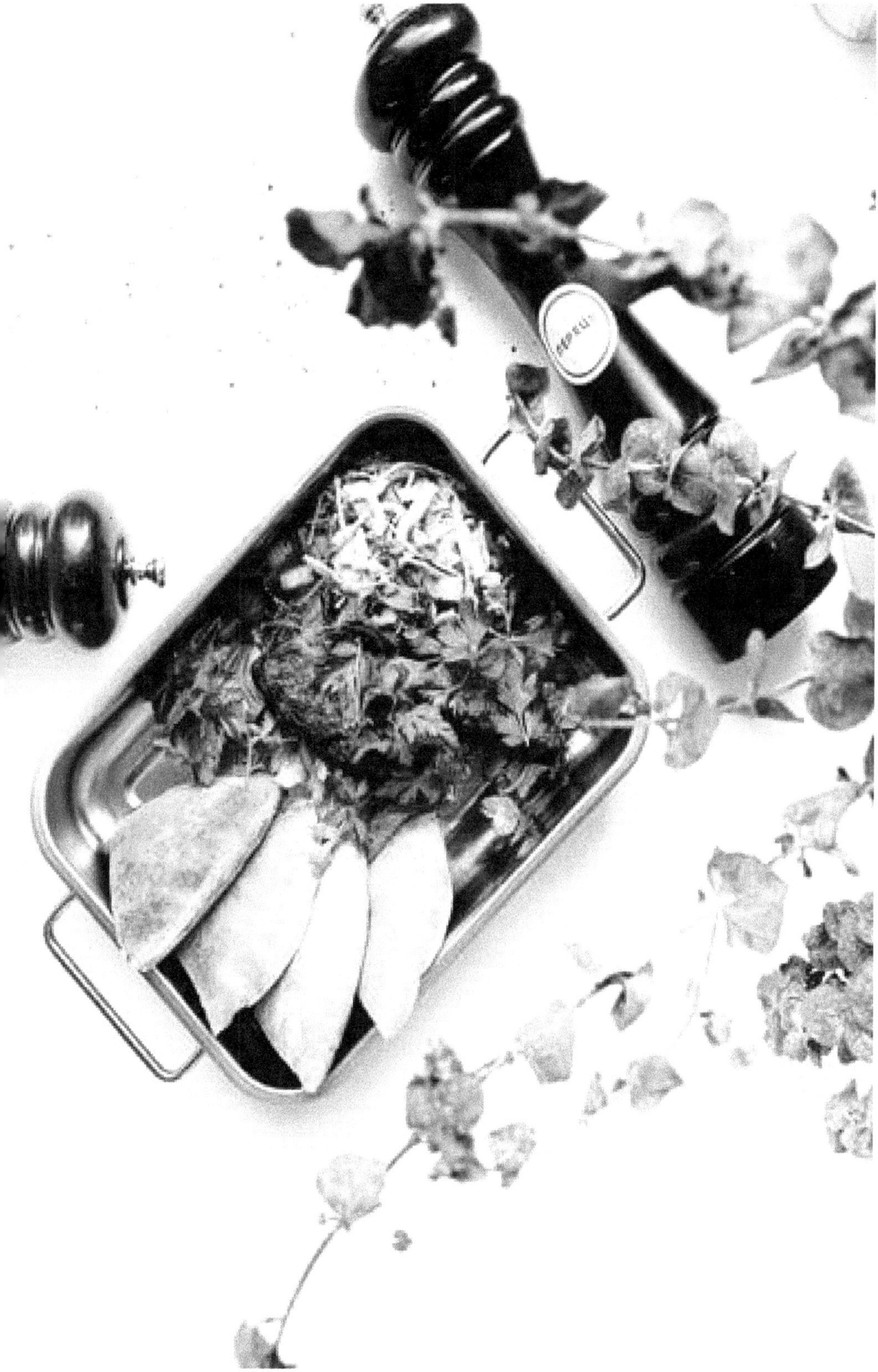

Creamy Mushroom and Kale

3 Servings

Preparation Time: 15 minutes

Ingredients

- 2 tbsps coconut oil
- 1 clove of garlic, minced
- 1 onion chopped up
- 1 bunch kale, stems removed and leaves chopped up
- 12 white button mushrooms chopped up
- 1 cup coconut milk
- Salt and pepper to taste

Directions

- Heat oil in a pan.
- Sauté the garlic and onion until fragrant for 2 minutes.
- Mix in mushrooms. Season with pepper and salt. Cook for 8 minutes.
- Mix in kale and coconut milk. Simmer for 5 minutes.
- Adjust seasoning to taste.

Crunchy Kale Chips

8 Servings

Preparation Time: 2 hours

Ingredients

- 2 tbsps filtered water
- ½ tbsp sea salt
- 1 tbsp raw honey
- 2 tbsps nutritional yeast
- 1 lemon, juiced
- 1 cup sweet potato, grated
- 1 cup fresh cashews soaked 2 hours
- 2 bunches green curly kale, washed, ribs and stems removed, leaves torn into bite-sized pieces

Directions

- Prepare a baking sheet by covering it with unbleached parchment paper. Preheat oven to 150of.
- In a large mixing bowl, place kale.
- In a food processor, process the remaining ingredients until smooth. Pour over kale.
- With your hands, coat kale with marinade.

- Evenly spread kale onto parchment paper and pop in the oven. Dehydrate for 2 hours and turn leaves after the first hour of baking.
- Remove from oven; let it cool completely before serving.

Delicious Roasted Eggplant

6 Servings

Preparation Time: 30 minutes

Ingredients

- Pinch of sugar
- ¼ tbsp salt
- ¼ tbsp cayenne pepper or to taste
- 1 tbsp parsley, flat leaf, and chopped up finely
- 2 tbsps fresh basil, chopped up
- 1 small chili pepper seeded and minced, optional
- ½ cup red onion, finely chopped up
- ½ cup Greek feta cheese, crushed
- ¼ cup extra virgin olive oil
- 2 tbsps lemon juice
- 1 medium eggplant, around 1 pound

Directions

- Preheat broiler and position rack 6 inches away from heat source.
- Pierce the eggplant with a knife or fork.
- Then with a foil, line a baking pan and place the eggplant and broil.

- Make sure to turn eggplant every five minutes or until the skin is charred and eggplant is soft, which takes around 14 to 18 minutes of broiling.
- Once done, remove from heat and let cool.
- In a medium bowl, add lemon.
- Then cut eggplant in half, lengthwise, and scrape the flesh, and place in the bowl with lemon.
- Add oil and mix until well combined.
- Then add salt, cayenne, parsley, basil, chili pepper, bell pepper, onion, and feta.
- Toss until well combined and add sugar to taste if wanted.

Tasty Stuffed Squash

4 Servings

Preparation Time: 30 minutes

Ingredients

- ¼ cup sour cream
- ½ cup shredded cheddar
- 1 tbsp taco sauce
- 1 small tomato chopped up
- ½ small green bell pepper seeded and chopped up
- ½ medium onion, chopped up
- 1 tbsp cumin
- 1 tbsp onion powder
- ¼ tbsp cayenne
- 1½ tbsps chili powder
- 1 can 15-ounce black beans, drained and rinsed
- 1 clove garlic, minced
- 1 tbsp olive oil
- 2 medium zucchinis
- 2 medium yellow squash
- Salt and pepper

Directions

- Boil until tender in a large pan of water, zucchini and yellow squash, then drain.
- Sideways, slice the squash and trim the ends. Take out the center flesh and chop.
- On medium-high level fire, place the skillet with oil and sauté garlic until fragrant.
- Add onion and tomato and sauté for 8 minutes. Add chopped-up squash, bell pepper, cumin, onion powder, cayenne, chili powder, and black beans, and continue cooking until veggies are tender.
- Season with pepper and salt to taste. Remove from fire.
- Spread 1 tbsp of taco sauce on each squash shell, fill with half of the cooked filling, top with cheese, and garnish with sour cream.
- Repeat procedure on other half of squash shell. Serve and enjoy.

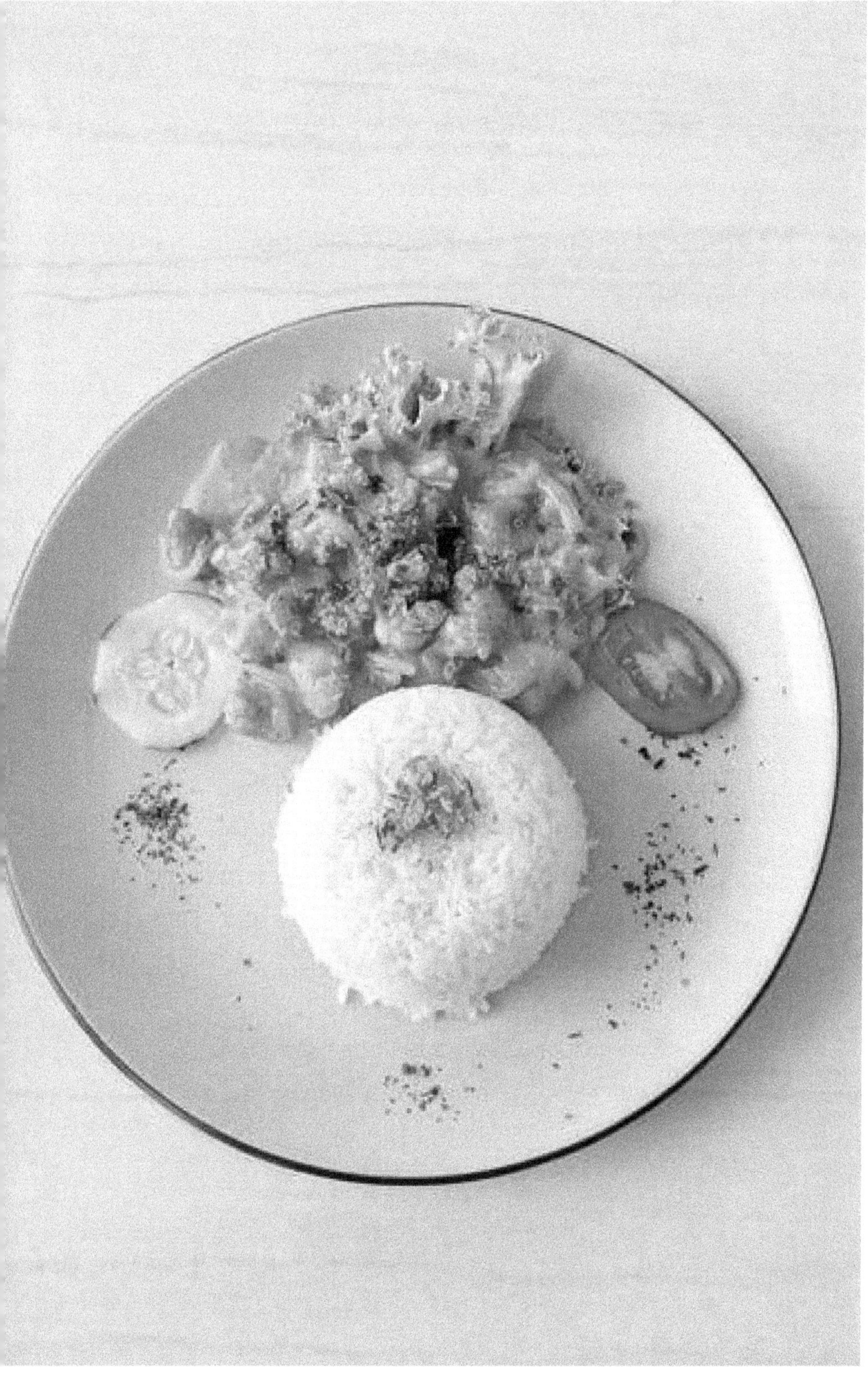

Colorful Baked Vegetables

6 Servings

Preparation Time: 1 hour and 15 minutes

Ingredients

- 2 pounds Brussels sprouts, trimmed
- 3 pounds Butternut squash, peeled, seeded, and cut into the same size as sprouts
- 1 pound pork breakfast sausage
- 1 tbsp fat from the fried sausage

Directions

- Grease a 9x13 inch baking pan and preheat the oven to 350°f.
- On medium high-level fire, place a large nonstick saucepan and cook sausage.
- Break up sausages and cook until browned.
- In a greased pan, mix browned sausage, squash, sprouts, sea salt, and fat.
- Toss to mix well.
- Pop into the oven and cook for an hour.
- Remove from oven and serve warm.

Cream and Carrot Chowder

8 Servings

Preparation Time: 40 minutes

Ingredients

- 8 fresh mint sprigs
- ½ cup 2% Greek-style plain yogurt
- 1 tbsp fresh ginger, peeled, and grated
- 2 cups chicken broth
- 1 pound. Baby carrots peeled and cut into 2-inch lengths
- 1/3 cup sliced shallots
- 2 tbsps sesame oil

Directions

- On medium fire, place a medium heavy bottom pan and heat oil.
- Sauté shallots until tender around 2 minutes.
- Add carrots and sauté for another 4 minutes.
- Pour broth, cover, and bring to a boil. Once the soup is boiling, slow fire to a simmer and cook carrots until tender around 22 minutes.
- Add ginger and continue cooking while covered for another eight minutes.
- Turn off the fire and let it cool for 10 minutes.

- Pour mixture into blender and puree. If needed, puree carrots in batches, then return to pan.
- Heat pureed carrots until heated through around 2 minutes.
- Turn off the fire and evenly pour into 8 serving bowls.
- Serve and enjoy, or you can store in the freezer in 8 different covered containers for a quick soup in the middle of the week.

BRUNCH

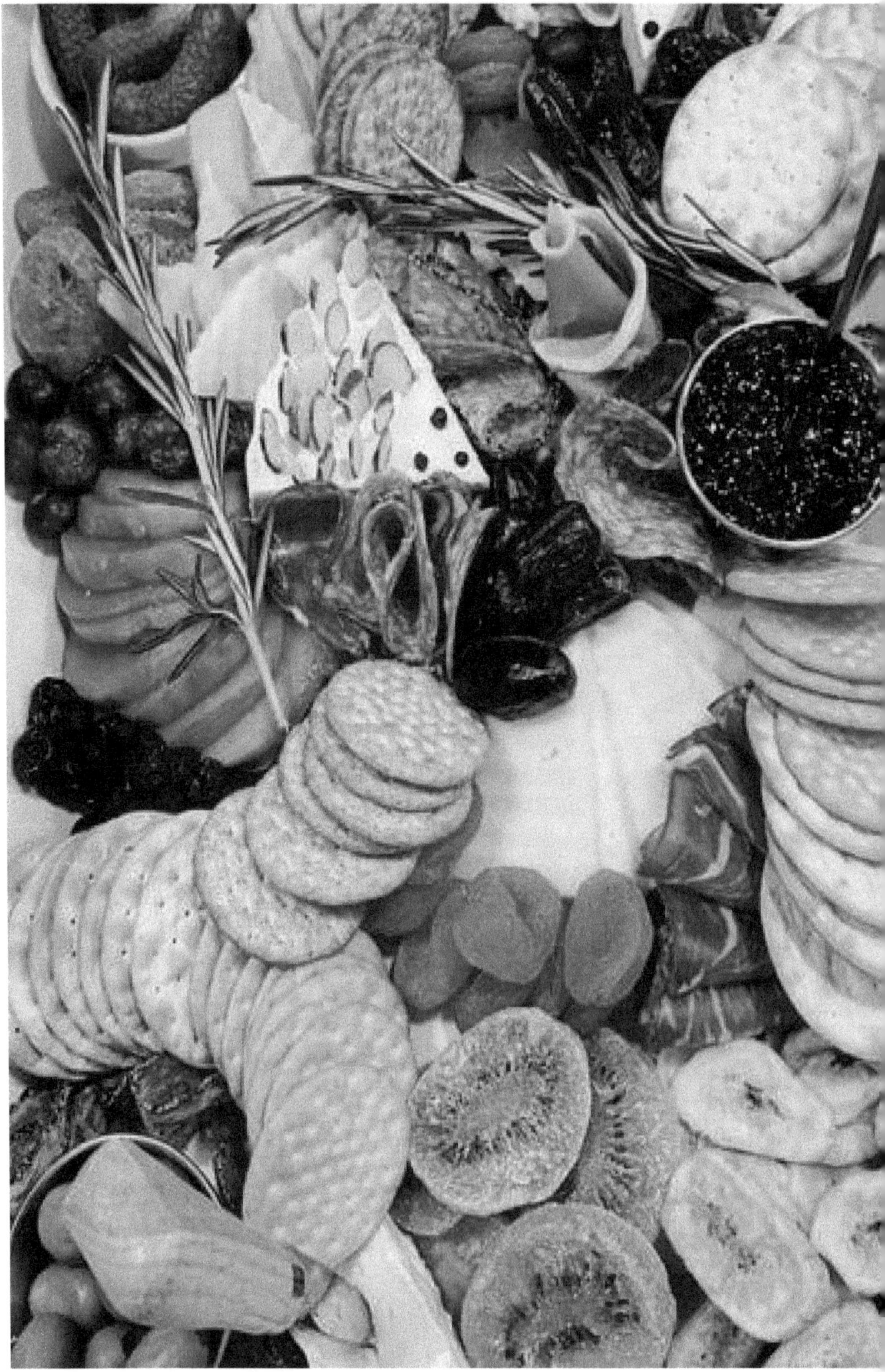

Eggs Benedict and Artichoke Hearts

2 Servings

Preparation Time: 30 minutes

Ingredients

- Salt and pepper to taste
- ¾ cup balsamic vinegar
- 4 artichoke hearts
- ¼ cup bacon, cooked
- 1 egg white
- 8 eggs
- 1 tbsp lemon juice
- ¾ cup melted ghee or butter

Directions

- Line a baking sheet with parchment paper or foil.
- Preheat the oven to 3750f.
- Deconstruct the artichokes and remove the hearts.
- Place the hearts in balsamic vinegar for 20 minutes.
- Set aside.
- Prepare the hollandaise sauce by using four eggs and separate the yolk from the white.

- Reserve the egg white for the artichoke hearts.
- Add the yolks and lemon juice and cook in a double boiler while constantly mixing to create a silky texture of the sauce.
- Add the oil and season with salt and pepper.
- Set aside.
- Remove the artichoke hearts from the balsamic vinegar marinade and place them on the cookie sheet.
- Brush the artichokes with the egg white and cook in the oven for 20 minutes.
- Poach the remaining four eggs.
- Turn up the heat and let the water boil.
- Crack the eggs one at a time and cook for a minute before removing the egg.
- Assemble by layering the artichokes, bacon, and poached eggs.
- Pour over the hollandaise sauce.
- Serve with toasted bread.

Eggs with Kale Hash

4 Servings

Preparation Time: 20 minutes

Ingredients

- 4 large eggs
- 1 bunch chopped kale
- 1 Dash of ground nutmeg
- 2 sweet potatoes, chopped up
- 1 or 14.5-ounce can of chicken broth

Directions

- In a large nonstick skillet, bring the chicken broth to a simmer.
- Add the sweet potatoes and season lightly with salt and pepper.
- Add a dash of nutmeg to improve the flavor.
- Cook until the sweet potatoes become soft, around 10 minutes.
- Add kale and season with salt and pepper.
- Continue cooking for four minutes or until kale has wilted.
- Set aside.
- Using the same skillet, heat 1 tbsp of olive oil over medium high-level heat.

- Cook the eggs sunny side up until the whites become opaque and the yolks have set.
- Top the kale hash with the eggs.
- Serve immediately.

Bacon Quiche

6 Servings

Preparation Time: 47 minutes

Ingredients
Topping ingredients

- 2 small, medium-sized tomatoes, sliced

Quiche ingredients

- ¼ tbsp black pepper
- ¼ tbsp salt
- ¼ tbsp ground mustard
- ½ cup fresh spinach, chopped up
- 2/4 cups cauliflower, ground into rice
- 5 slices nitrate-free bacon cooked and chopped up
- 2 tbsps unsweetened plain almond milk
- ½ cup organic white eggs
- 6 eggs, beaten.

Zucchini hash crust:

- 1/8 tbsp sea salt
- 1 tbsp butter
- 1 tbsp flax meal
- 1 ½ tbsp coconut flour
- 1 egg, beaten

- 2 smalls to medium sized organic zucchini, grated

Directions

- Grease a pie dish and preheat the oven to 400of.
- Grate zucchini, drain, and squeeze dry.
- In a bowl, add dry zucchini and remaining crust ingredients and mix well.
- Place in the bottom of the pie plate and press down as if making a pie crust.
- Pop in the oven and bake for 9 minutes.
- Meanwhile, in a large mixing bowl, whisk well black pepper, salt, mustard, almond milk, egg whites, and egg.
- Add bacon, spinach, and cauliflower rice. Mix well. Pour into baked zucchini crust, top with tomato slices.
- Pop back in the oven and bake for 28 minutes. If at 20 minutes baking time top is browning too much, cover with parchment paper for the remainder of cooking time.
- Once done cooking, remove from oven, let it stand for at least ten minutes.
- Slice into equal triangles, serve and enjoy.

Crispy Potato Rosti

4 Servings

Preparation Time: 15 minutes

Ingredients

- ½ pound russet potatoes peeled and grated roughly
- Salt and freshly ground black pepper, to taste
- 3.5 ounces smoked salmon cut into slices
- 1 tsp olive oil
- 1 tbsp chives chopped up finely
- 2 tbsps sour cream

Directions

- Preheat the air fryer to 360 degrees f and grease a pizza pan with the olive oil.
- Add chives, potatoes, salt, and black pepper in a large bowl and mix until well combined.
- Place the potato mixture into the prepared pizza pan and pour the pizza pan in an air fryer basket.
- Cook for about 15 minutes and cut the potato rosti into pieces.
- Top with the smoked salmon slices and sour cream and serve.

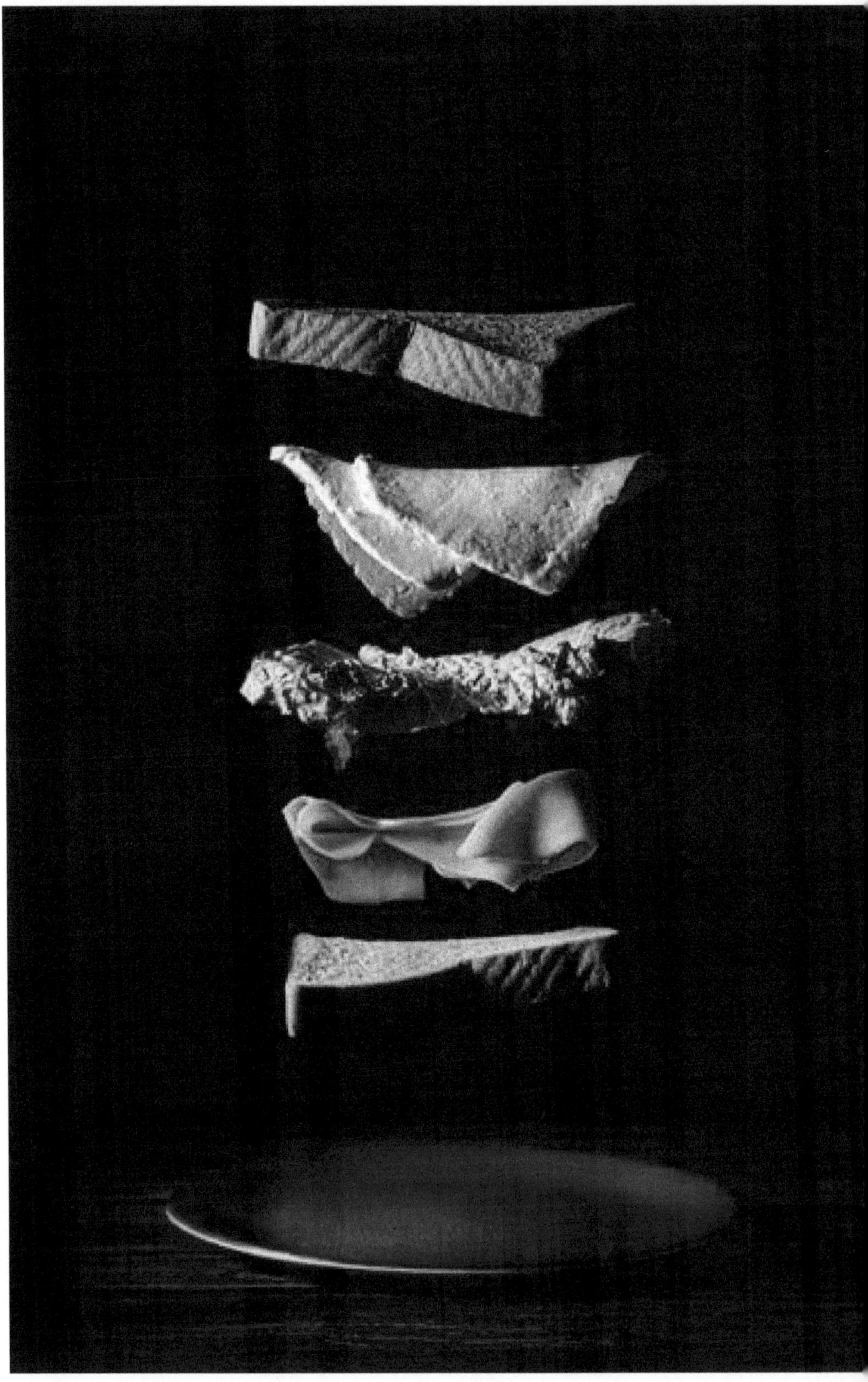

Classical Pumpkin Pancakes

8 Servings

Preparation Time: 20 minutes

Ingredients

- 2 squares puff pastry
- 6 tbsps pumpkin filling
- 2 small eggs, beaten
- ¼ tsp cinnamon

Directions

- Preheat the air fryer to 360 degrees f and roll out a square of puff pastry.
- Layer it with pumpkin pie filling, leaving about ¼-inch space around the edges.
- Cut it up into equal-sized square pieces and cover the gaps with beaten egg.
- Arrange the squares into a baking dish and cook for about 12 minutes.
- Sprinkle some cinnamon and serve.

Easy Cheese Sandwiches

4 Servings

Preparation Time: 10 minutes

Ingredients

- 8 American cheese slices
- 8 bread slices
- 8 tsps butter

Directions

- Preheat the air fryer to 365 degrees f and arrange cheese slices between bread slices.
- Spread butter over the outer sides of the sandwich and repeat with the remaining butter, slices, and cheese.
- Arrange the sandwiches in an air fryer basket and cook for about 8 minutes, flipping once in the middle way.

Vegetable Mix Fry with Fresh Ginger

4 Servings

Preparation Time: 5 minutes

Ingredients

- 1 tbsp oil
- 2 cloves of garlic, minced
- 1 onion chopped up
- 1 thumb-size ginger, sliced
- 1 tbsp water
- 1 large carrot peeled and julienned
- 1 large green bell pepper seeded and julienned
- 1 large yellow bell pepper seeded and julienned
- 1 large red bell pepper seeded and julienned
- 1 zucchini, julienned
- Salt and pepper to taste

Directions

- Heat oil in a skillet over medium flame and sauté the garlic, onion, and ginger until fragrant.
- Mix in the rest of the ingredients and adjust the flame to a high level.

- Keep on mixing for at least 5 minutes until vegetables are half-cooked.
- Place in individual containers.
- Put a label and store it in the fridge.
- Let thaw at room temperature before heating in the microwave oven.

Eggplant Caprese

4 Servings

Preparation Time: 20 minutes

Ingredients

- 1 eggplant aubergine, small/medium
- 1 tomato large
- 2 basil leaves or a little more as needed
- 4-ounce mozzarella
- Good quality olive oil
- Pepper and salt to taste

Directions

- Cut the ends of the eggplant and then cut it lengthwise into ¼-inch thick slices.
- Discard the smaller pieces that are mostly skin and short.
- Slice the tomatoes and mozzarella into thin slices just like the eggplant.
- On the fire to medium-high level, place a griddle and let it heat up.
- Brush eggplant slices with olive oil and place on grill.
- Grill for 3 minutes.
- Turn over and grill for a minute.

- Add a slice of cheese on one side and tomato on the other side.
- Continue cooking for another 2 minutes.
- Sprinkle with basil leaves.
- Season with pepper and salt.
- Fold eggplant in half and skewer with a cocktail stick.
- Serve and enjoy.

Grilled Cheese Sandwich with Zucchini Bread

2 Servings

Preparation Time: 40 minutes

Ingredients

- 1 large egg
- ½ cup freshly grated parmesan
- ¼ cup almond flour
- 2 cups grated zucchini
- 2 cups shredded cheddar
- 2 green onions finely sliced
- Freshly ground black pepper
- Kosher salt
- Vegetable oil, for cooking

Directions

- With a paper towel, squeeze dries the zucchinis and place in a bowl.
- Add almond flour, green onions, parmesan, and egg.
- Season with pepper and salt.
- Whisk well to combine.
- Place a large nonstick pan on medium fire and add oil to the cover pan.

- Once hot, add ¼ cup of zucchini mixture and shape into a square like bread.
- Add another batch as many as you can put in the pan.
- If needed, cook in batches.
- Cook for four minutes per side and place on a paper towel-lined plate.
- Once done cooking zucchinis, wipe off the oil from the pan.
- Place one zucchini piece on the pan; spread ½ of shredded cheese, and then top with another piece of zucchini.
- Grill for two minutes per side.
- Repeat the process to make 2 sandwiches.
- Serve and enjoy.

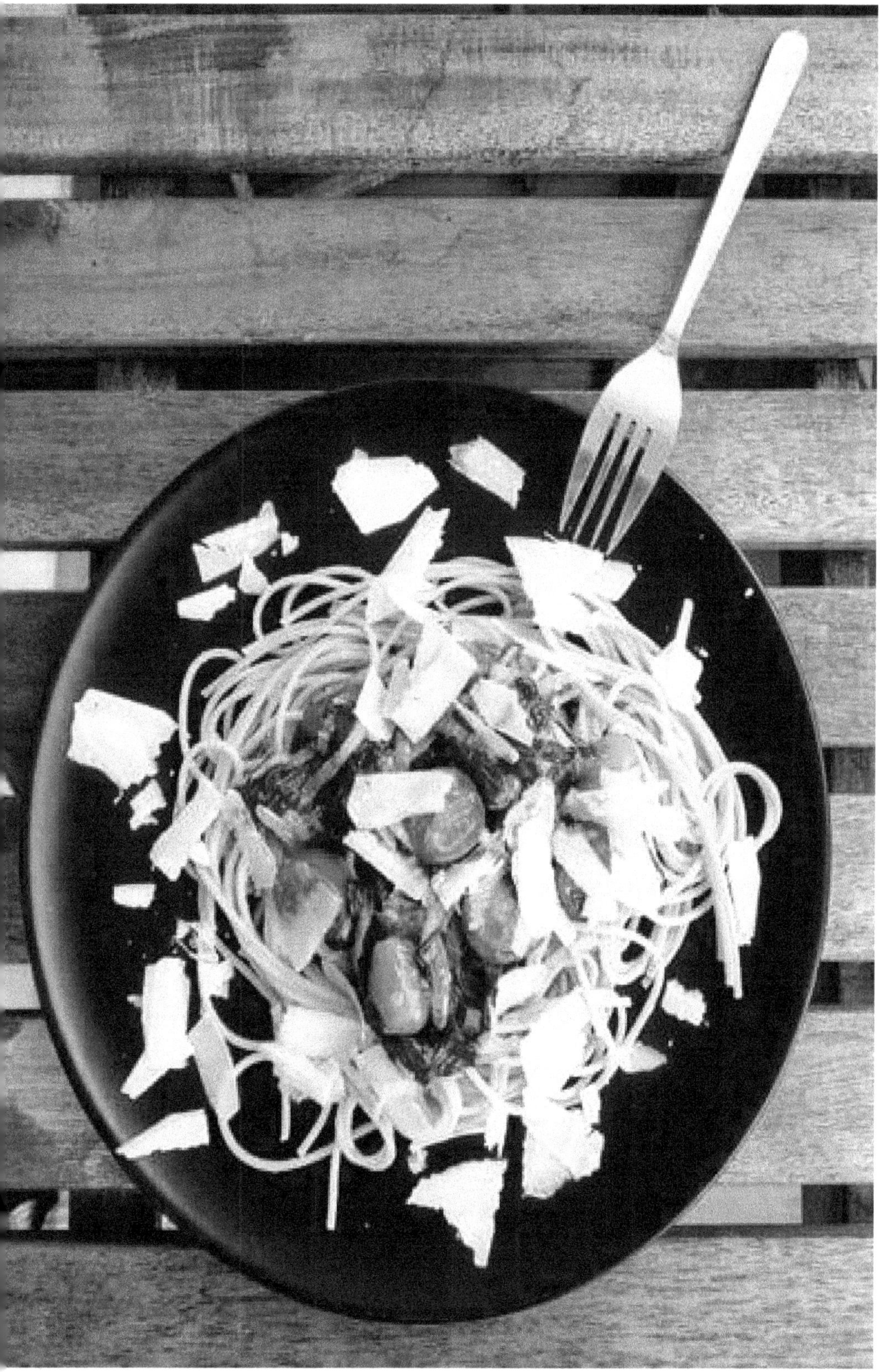

Standard Quiche

6 Servings

Preparation Time: 46 minutes

Ingredients

- 4-ounce sliced portobello mushrooms
- Pepper and salt to taste
- ½ tbsp dried basil
- ½ tbsp dried parsley
- 6 eggs, whisked
- ¾ pound pork breakfast sausage

Directions

- Grease a 9-inch round pie plate or baking pan and preheat the oven to 350°f.
- On medium fire, place a nonstick fry pan and cook sausage.
- Mix fry until cooked as you break them into pieces.
- Discard excess oil once cooked.
- In a big bowl, whisk pepper, salt, basil, parsley, and eggs.
- Pour into prepped baking plate.

- Pop into the oven and bake until the middle is firm, around 30-35 minutes.
- Once done, remove from oven; let it stand for 10 minutes before slicing and serving.

DINNER

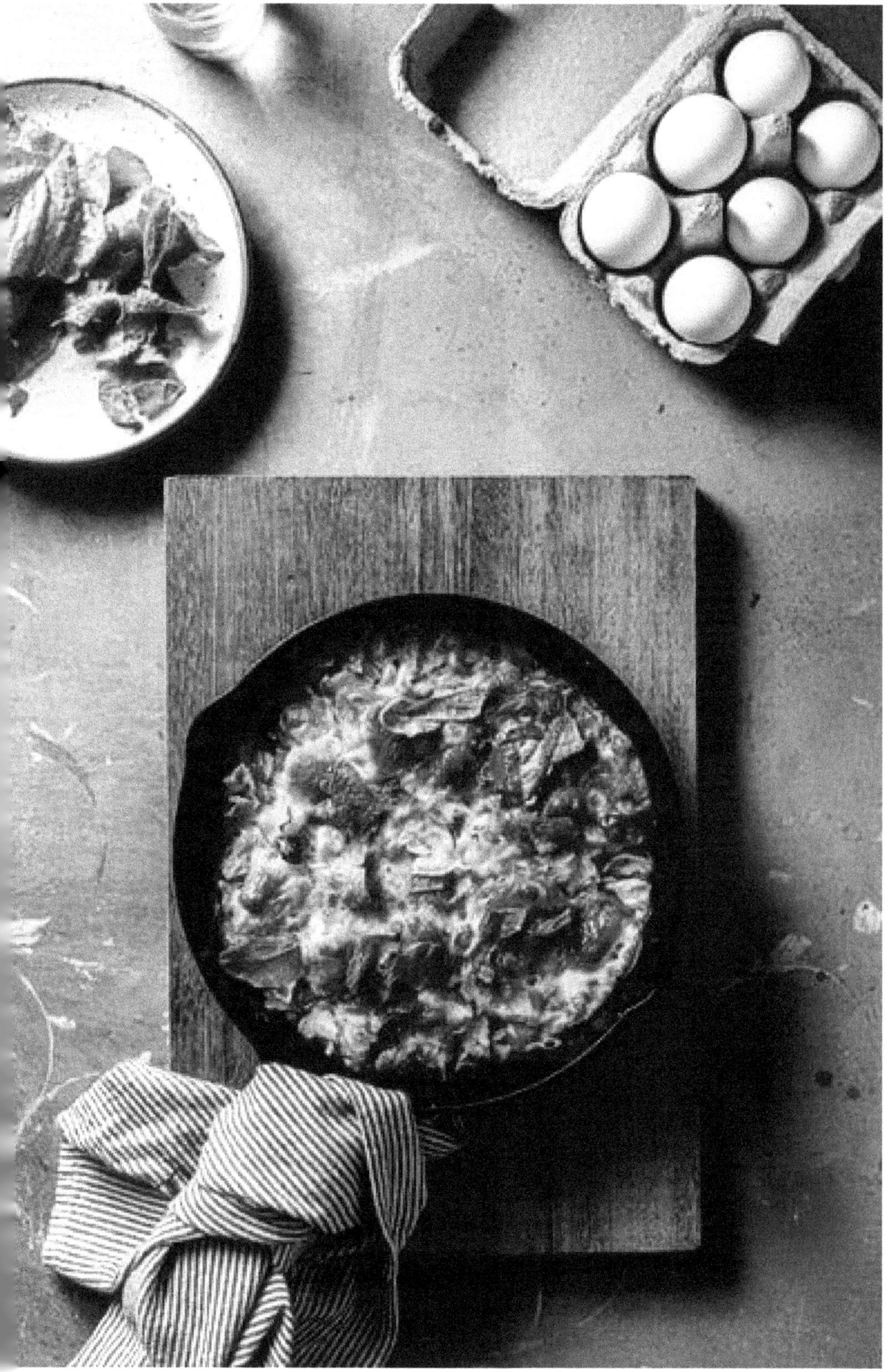

Tangy Zucchini Tomato Frittata

8 Servings

Preparation Time: 30 minutes

Ingredients

- 3 pounds tomatoes finely sliced crosswise
- ¾ cup cheddar cheese, shredded
- ¼ cup milk
- 8 large eggs
- 1 tbsp fresh thyme leaves
- 3 zucchinis cut into ¼-inch thick rounds
- 1 onion finely chopped up
- 1 tbsp olive oil
- Salt and pepper to taste

Directions

- Preheat the oven to 425 degrees Fahrenheit.
- Prepare a nonstick skillet and heat it over medium heat.
- Sauté the zucchini, onion, and thyme.
- Cook and mix often for 8 to 10 minutes.
- Let the liquid in the pan evaporate and season with salt and pepper to taste.
- Remove the skillet from heat.

- In a bowl, whisk the milk, cheese, eggs, salt, and pepper together.
- Pour the egg mixture over the zucchini in the skillet.
- Lift the zucchini to let the eggs to coat the pan. Arrange the tomato slices on top.
- Return to the skillet and heat to medium-low fire and cook until the sides are set or golden brown, around 7 minutes.
- Place the skillet inside the oven and cook for 10 to 15 minutes or until the center of the frittata is cooked through.
- To check if the egg is cooked through, insert a wooden skewer in the middle, and it should come out clean.
- Remove from the oven and loosen the frittata from the skillet. Serve warm.

Indian style Bell Peppers and Potato Mix

2 Servings

Preparation Time: 15 minutes

Ingredients

- 1 tbsp oil
- ½ tsp cumin seeds
- 2 cloves of garlic, minced
- Potatoes, scrubbed and cut in halves
- Salt and pepper to taste
- Tbsps water
- 2 bell peppers seeded and julienned
- Chopped up cilantro for garnish

Directions

- Heat oil in a skillet over medium flame and toast the cumin seeds until fragrant.
- Add the garlic until fragrant.
- Mix in the potatoes, salt, pepper, water, and bell peppers.
- Close the cover and let simmer for at least 10 minutes.
- Garnish with cilantro before cooking time ends.

- Place in individual containers.
- Put a label and store it in the fridge.
- Let thaw at room temperature before heating in the microwave oven.

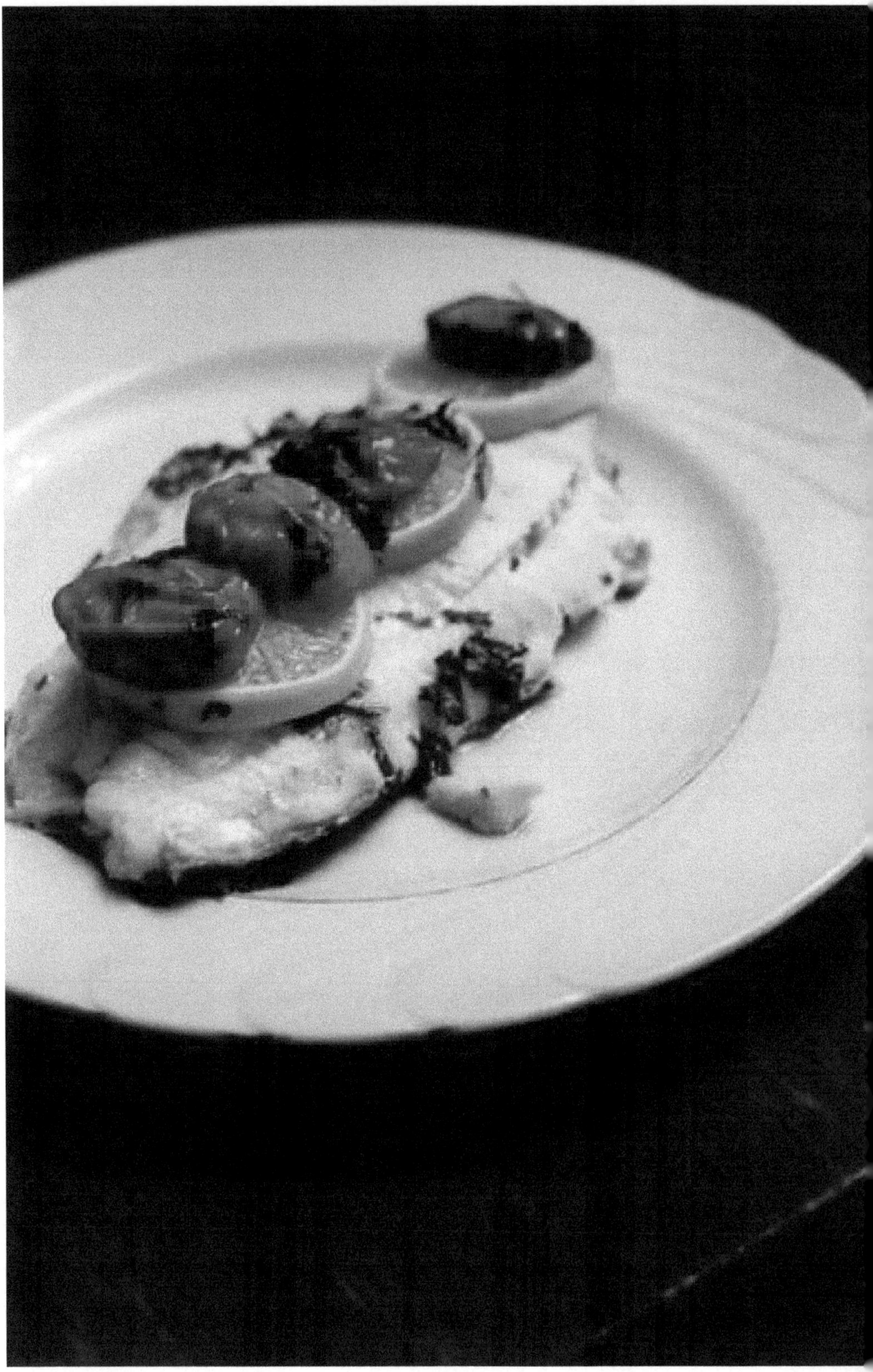

Greek Savory Veggie-Rice

6 Servings

Preparation Time: 20 minutes

Ingredients

- Pepper and salt to taste
- ¼ cup extra virgin olive oil
- 1 tbsp chopped up fresh mint
- ½ cup grape tomatoes, cut in halves
- ½ red bell pepper, diced small
- 1 head cauliflower cut into large florets
- ¼ cup fresh lemon juice
- ½ yellow onion, minced

Directions

- In a bowl, mix lemon juice and onion and leave for 30 minutes.
- Drain onion and reserve the juice and onion bits.
- In a blender, shred cauliflower until the size of a grain of rice.
- On medium fire, place a medium nonstick skillet, and for 8-10 minutes, cook cauliflower while covered.

- Add grape tomatoes and bell pepper and cook for 3 minutes while mixing occasionally.
- Add mint and onion bits.
- Cook for another three minutes.
- Meanwhile, in a small bowl, whisk pepper, salt, 3 tbsps reserved lemon juice, and olive oil until well blended.
- Remove cooked cauliflower, pour to a serving bowl, pour lemon juice mixture, and toss to mix.
- Before serving, if needed, season with pepper and salt to taste.

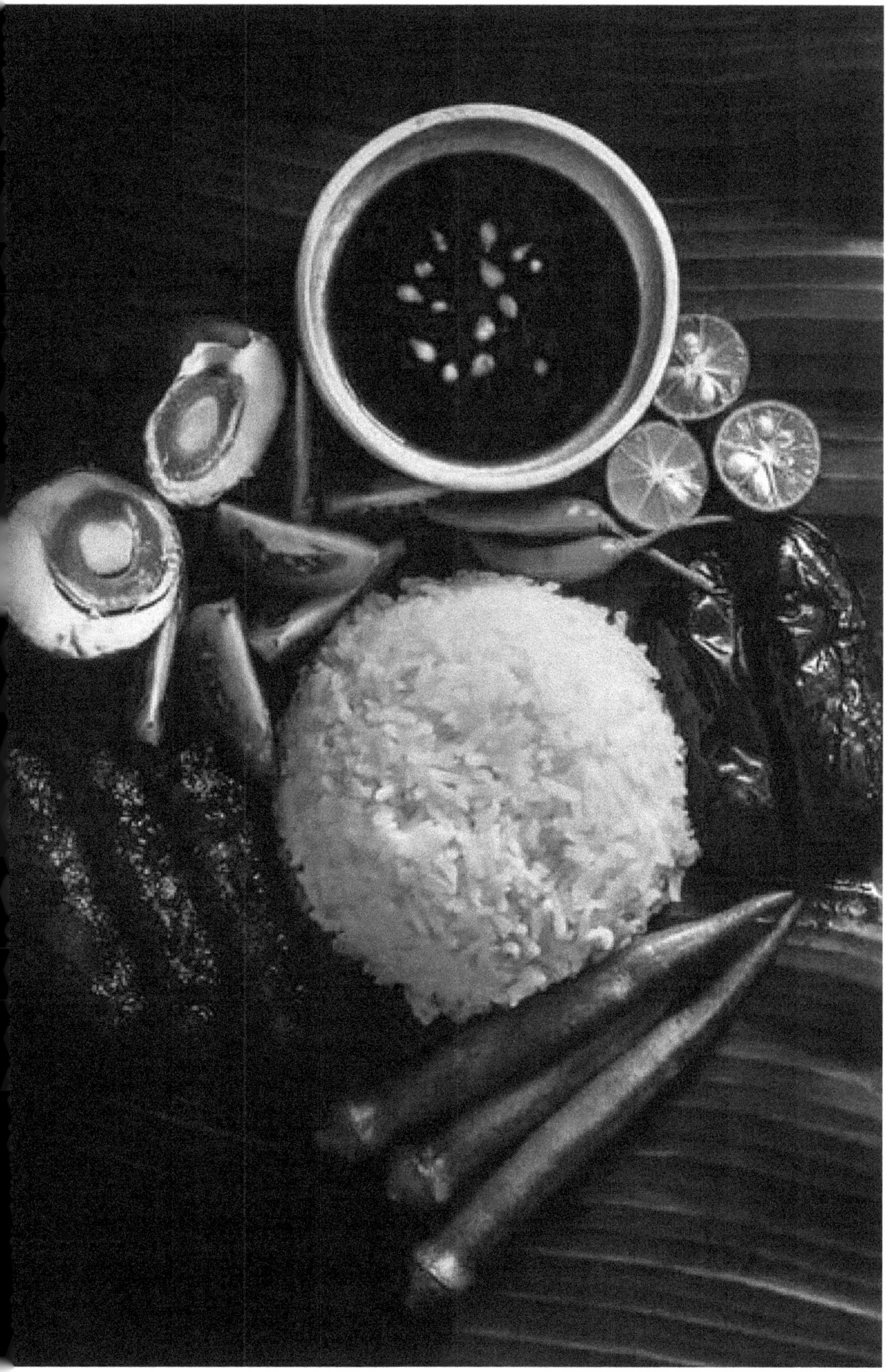

Zucchini Noodles with Eggplant Bolognese

4 Servings

Preparation Time: 20 minutes

Ingredients

- 6 leaves of fresh basil chopped up
- 1 or 28-ounce can plum tomatoes
- ½ cup red wine
- 1 tbsp tomato paste
- sprigs of thyme chopped up
- 2 bay leaves
- 2 cloves garlic, minced
- 1 large yellow onion chopped up
- Salt and pepper to taste
- 2 tbsps extra-virgin olive oil
- ½ pound ground beef
- 1½ pounds eggplant, diced
- 2 cups zucchini noodles

Directions

- Heat the skillet over medium high-level heat and add oil.
- Sauté the onion and beef and sprinkle with salt and pepper.
- Sauté for 10 minutes until the meat is brown.

- Add in the eggplants, bay leaves, garlic, and thyme.
- Cook for another 15 minutes.
- Once the eggplant is tender, add the tomato paste and wine.
- Add the tomatoes and crush using a spoon.
- Bring to a boil and reduce the heat to low.
- Simmer for 10 minutes.
- In a skillet, add oil and sauté the zucchini noodles for five minutes.
- Turn off the heat.
- Pour the tomato sauce over the zucchini noodles and garnish with fresh basil.

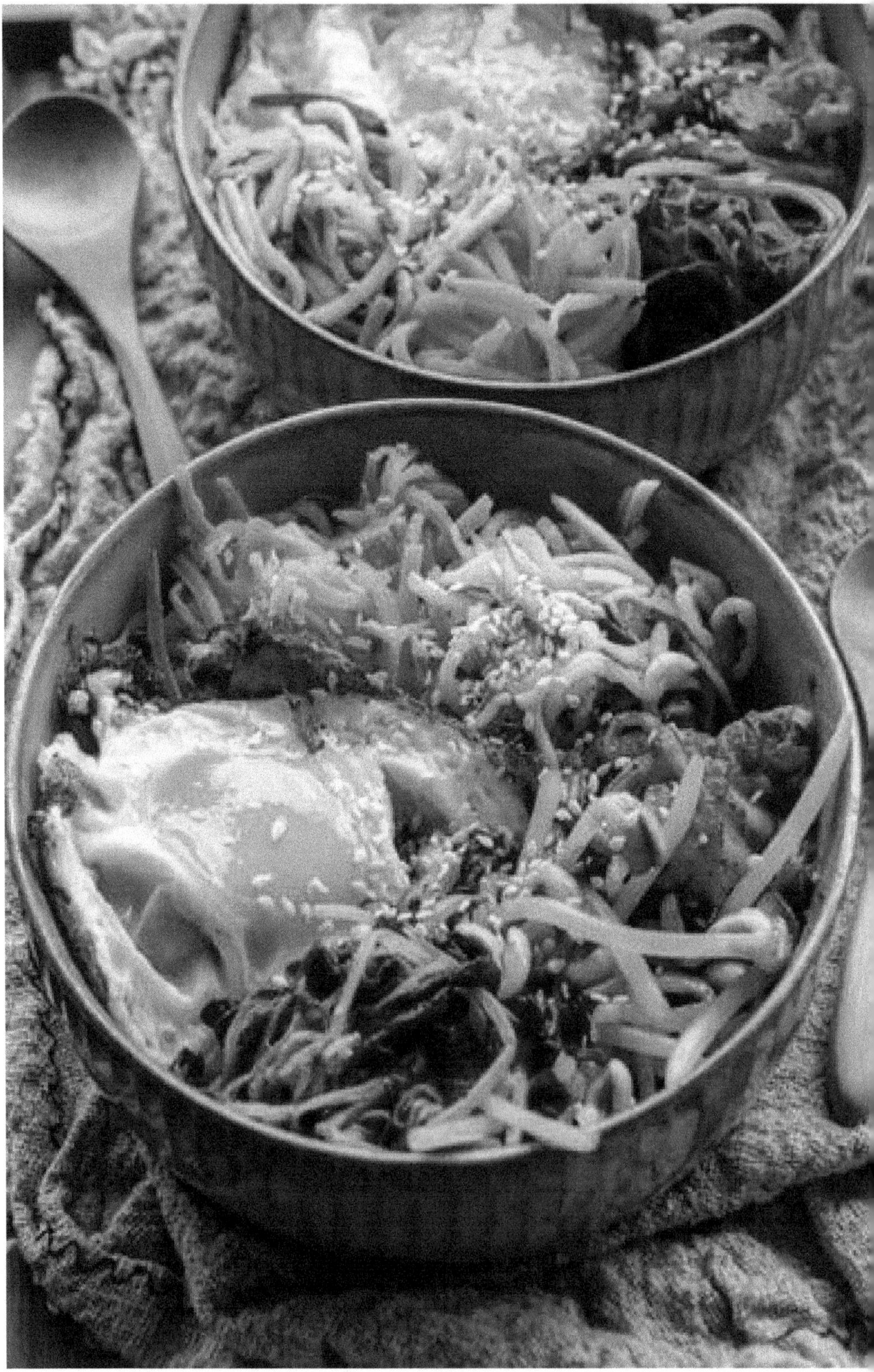

Feta Cheese and Roast Eggplant Dip

12 Servings

Preparation Time: 20 minutes

Ingredients

- ¼ tbsp salt
- ¼ tbsp cayenne pepper
- 1 tbsp finely chopped up flat-leaf parsley
- 2 tbsps chopped up fresh basil
- 1 small chile pepper
- 1 small red bell pepper finely chopped up
- ½ cup finely chopped up red onion
- ½ cup crushed Greek nonfat feta cheese
- ¼ cup extra-virgin olive oil
- 2 tbsps lemon juice
- 1 medium eggplant, around 1 pound

Directions

- Preheat broiler, position rack on the top-most part of the oven, and line a baking pan with foil.
- With a fork or knife, poke eggplant, place on the prepared baking pan, and broil for 5 minutes per side until skin is charred all around.

- Once eggplant skin is charred, remove from broiler, and let cool to handle.
- Once the eggplant is cool enough to handle, slice in half lengthwise, scoop out the flesh, and place in a medium bowl.
- Pour in lemon juice and toss eggplant to coat with lemon juice and prevent it from discoloring.
- Add oil; continue mixing until oil is absorbed by the eggplant.
- Mix in salt, cayenne pepper, parsley, basil, chile pepper, bell pepper, onion, and feta.
- Toss to mix well and serve.

Sour Cream with Garlic Zucchini Bake

3 Servings

Preparation Time: 20 minutes

Ingredients

- 1 Quarter cup grated parmesan cheese
- Paprika to taste
- 1 tbsp minced garlic
- 1 large zucchini cut lengthwise then in half
- 1 cup sour cream
- 1 package cream cheese, softened

Directions

- Lightly grease a casserole dish with cooking spray.
- Place zucchini slices in a single layer in the dish.
- In a bowl, whisk well, remaining ingredients except for paprika.
- Spread on top of zucchini slices.
- Sprinkle paprika.
- Cover dish with foil.
- For 10 minutes, cook in a preheated 390-degree oven.
- Remove foil and cook for 10 minutes. Serve and enjoy.

Rosemary with Garlic Potatoes

4 Servings

Preparation Time: 2 minutes

Ingredients

- 1-pound potatoes peeled and sliced finely
- 2 garlic cloves
- ½ tsp salt
- 1 tbsp olive oil
- 2 sprigs of rosemary

Directions

- Place a trivet or steamer basket in the instant pan and pour in a cup of water.
- In a baking dish that can fit inside the instant pan, combine all ingredients, and toss to coat everything.
- Cover the baking dish with aluminum foil and place it on the steamer basket.
- Close the cover and press the steam button.
- Adjust the cooking time to 30 minutes.
- Do quick pressure release.
- Once cooled, evenly divide into serving size, keep in your preferred container, and refrigerate until ready to eat.

Tangy Mushroom Frittata

8 Servings

Preparation Time: 8 minutes

Ingredients

- ¼ cup mushroom, sliced
- 10 eggs
- 1 cup cherry tomatoes
- Salt
- Pepper
- 1 tsp olive oil

Directions

- Whisk the eggs in a bowl.
- Add the eggs into a skillet.
- Add the mushroom, cherry tomatoes and season using salt and pepper.
- Cover with cover and cook for about 5 to 8 minutes on low heat.

Turmeric with Mushroom, Spinach Frittata

6 Servings

Preparation Time: 35 minutes

Ingredients

- ½ tbsp pepper
- ½ tbsp salt
- 1 tbsp turmeric
- 5-ounce firm tofu
- 2 large eggs
- 6 large egg whites
- ¼ cup water
- 1-pound fresh spinach
- 6 cloves freshly chopped up garlic
- 1 large onion chopped up
- 1 pound button mushrooms, sliced

Directions

- Grease a 10-inch nonstick and oven-proof skillet and preheat the oven to 350of.
- Place skillet on medium high-level fire and add mushrooms.
- Cook until golden brown.
- Add onions, cook for 3 minutes, or until onions are tender.

- Add garlic, sauté for 30 seconds.
- Add water and spinach, cook while covered until spinach is wilted, around 2 minutes.
- Remove cover and continue cooking until water is fully evaporated.
- In a blender, puree pepper, salt, turmeric, tofu, eggs, and egg whites until smooth.
- Pour into skillet once the liquid is fully evaporated.
- Pop skillet into oven and bake until the center is set around 25-30 minutes.
- Remove skillet from oven and let it stand for ten minutes before inverting and pouring to a serving plate.
- Cut into 6 equal pieces, serve, and enjoy.

Smoked Salmon with Scrambled Eggs

1 Serving

Preparation Time: 8 minutes

Ingredients

- 1 tbsp coconut oil
- Pepper and salt to taste
- 1/8 tbsp red pepper flakes
- 1/8 tbsp garlic powder
- 1 tbsp fresh dill, chopped up finely
- 1 ounce smoked salmon, torn apart
- 2 whole eggs + 1 egg yolk, whisked

Directions

- In a big bowl, whisk the eggs. Mix in pepper, salt, red pepper flakes, garlic, dill, and salmon.
- On low fire, place a nonstick fry pan and lightly grease with oil.
- Pour egg mixture and whisk around until cooked through to make scrambled eggs, around 8 minutes on medium fire.
- Serve and enjoy.

Sausage, Spinach, Mushroom Frittata

4 Servings

Preparation Time: 30 minutes

Ingredients

- Salt and pepper to taste
- 10 eggs
- ½ small onions, chopped up
- 1 cup mushroom, sliced
- 1 cup fresh spinach chopped up
- ½ pound sausage, ground
- 2 tbsps coconut oil

Directions

- Preheat the oven to 350^0f.
- Heat a skillet over a medium high-level flame and add the coconut oil.
- Sauté the onions until softened. Add in the sausage and cook for two minutes.
- Add in the spinach and mushroom. Mix constantly until the spinach has wilted.
- Turn off the stove and distribute the vegetable mixture evenly.

- Pour in the beaten eggs and pour to the oven.
- Cook for twenty minutes or until the eggs are completely cooked through.

DESSERT

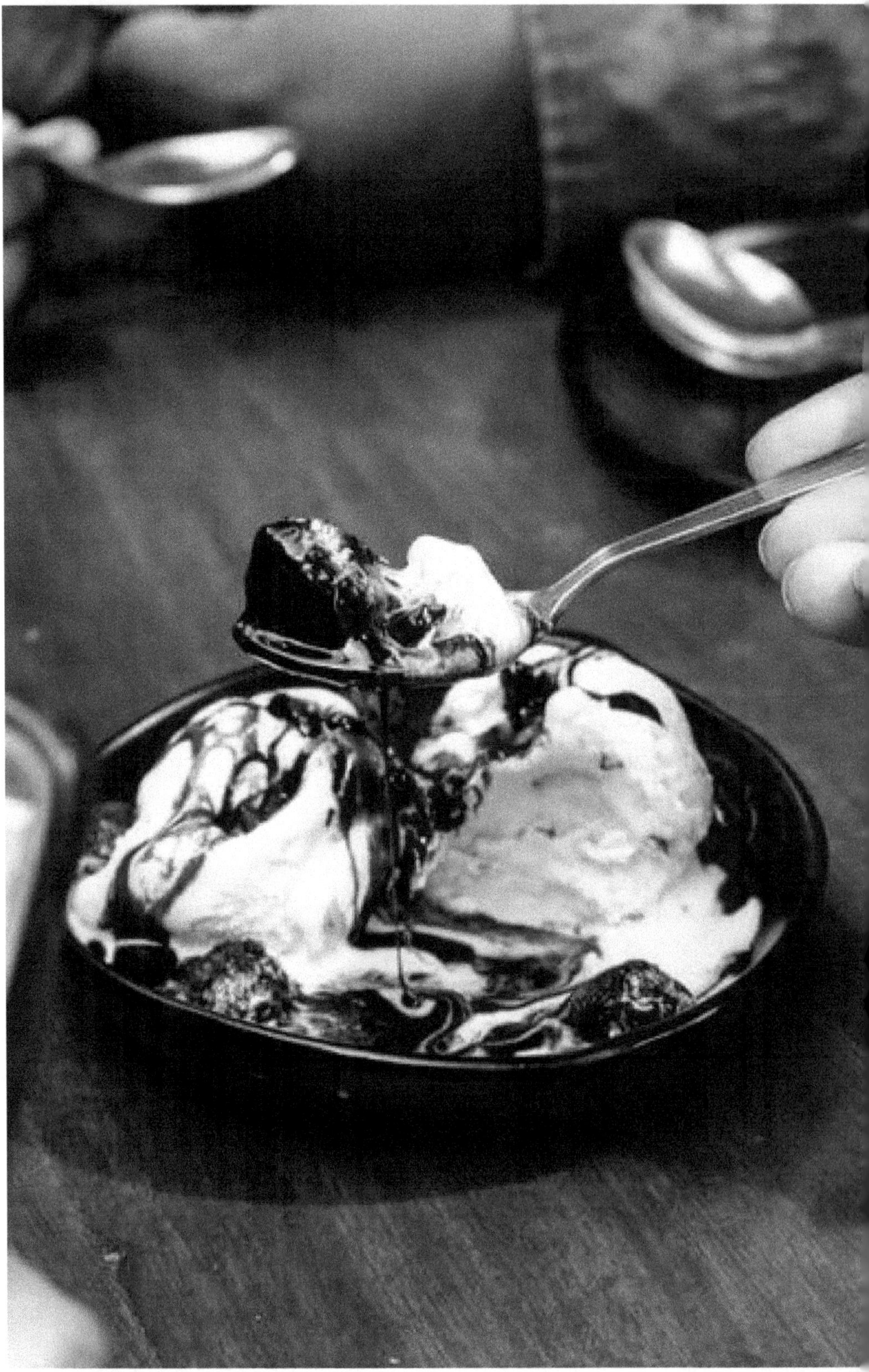

Macadamia Cold Cream

6 Servings

Preparation Time: 3 hours 40 minutes

Ingredients

- 1 tsp salt
- 3 eggs yolks
- 1 cup powdered sugar
- 1 cup chopped macadamia nuts
- 3 cups heavy cream
- 1½ tbsps sugar
- 1 cup macadamia butter, softened
- 1½ tbsps olive oil

Directions

- In a small pan, melt the heavy cream with macadamia butter, olive oil, sugar, and salt over low heat without boiling for about 3 minutes. Remove from the heat when it melts.
- Whisk the egg yolks in a bowl until creamy in color.
- Add the eggs into the cream mixture.

- Continue stirring until a thick batter has formed; about 3 minutes. Pour the cream mixture into a bowl.
- Refrigerate for 30 minutes, and add in the powdered sugar.
- Put the mixture into the ice cream machine and whip it accordingly.
- Add in the pecans after and spoon the mixture into a loaf pan.
- Freeze for 2 hours before serving.

Classic Cardamom Cookies

6 Servings

Preparation Time: 25 minutes

Ingredients

- 1 cup sugar
- 1 tsp salt
- 3 cups flour
- 1 cup butter, softened
- ¼ tsp baking soda

Coating:
- 2 tbsps sugar
- 1 tsp cardamom

Directions

- In a bowl, mix flour, butter, baking soda, sugar, and salt.
- Make balls out of the mixture and flatten them with your hands.
- Mix the cardamom and remaining sugar.
- Dip the cookies in the cardamom mixture and arrange them on a lined cookie sheet.
- Cook in the oven for about 15 minutes at 350ºF, until crispy.

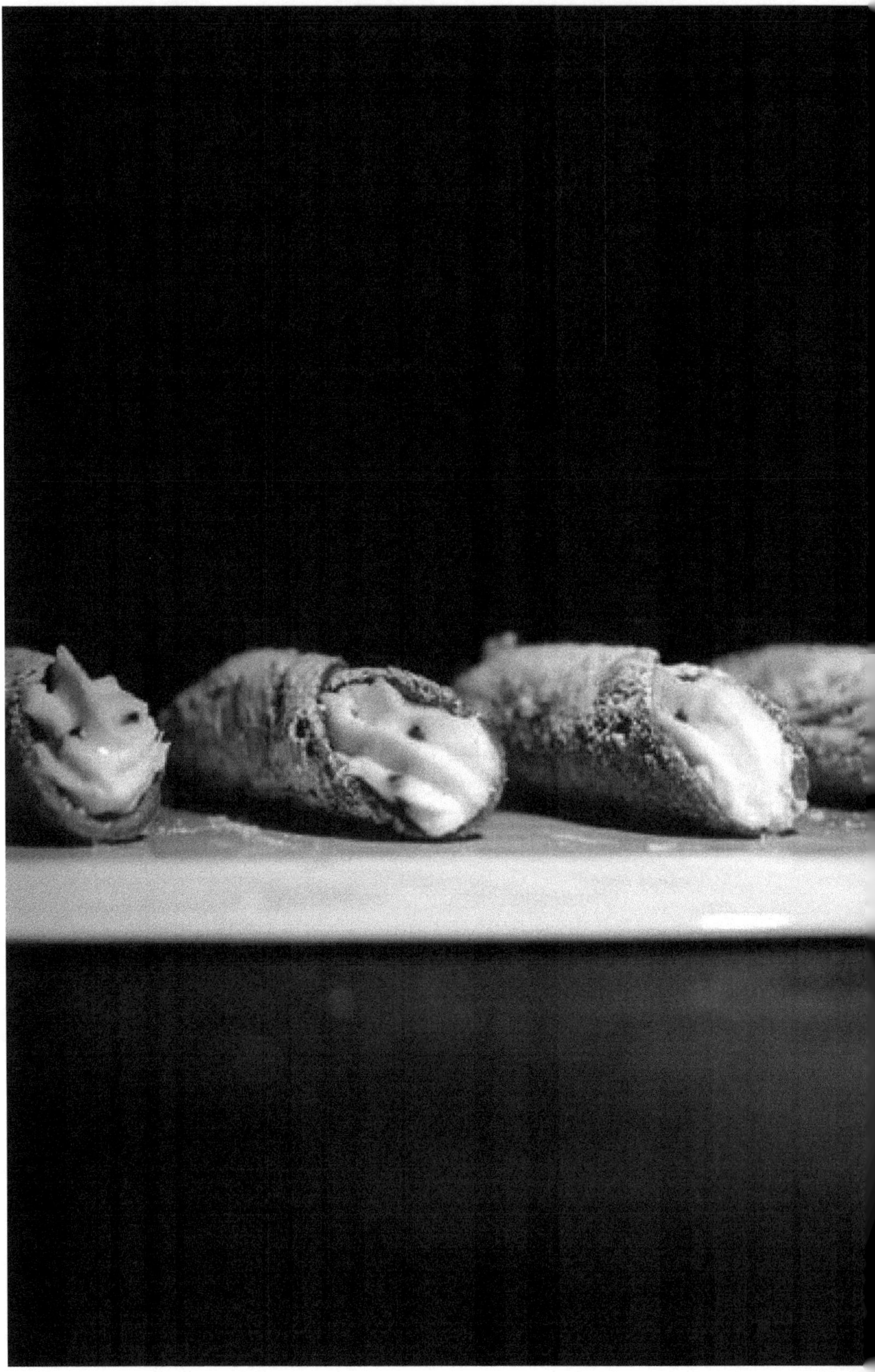

Cashew Nuts Cakes

8 Servings

Preparation Time: 25 minutes

Ingredients

- 1 tsp baking soda
- 1½ tbsp olive oil
- 24 walnuts halves
- 2 egg
- 2½ cups ground cashew
- 1 cup sugar

Directions

- Combine egg, ground cashew, baking soda, sugar, and olive oil, in a bowl and mix well.
- Make 20 balls out of the mixture and press them with your thumb onto a lined cookie sheet.
- Top each cookie with a half walnut. Bake for about 12 minutes at 350ºF.

American Style Chocolate Cheesecakes

6 Servings

Preparation Time: 4 min + cooling time

Ingredients

- 1 cup granulated sugar
- 1½ tsp vanilla extract
- 1 cup sour cream
- 2 cups mini dark chocolate chips
- 24 oz mascarpone, at time temperature

Directions

- Melt the chocolate with sour cream in the microwave for about 1 minute.
- Whisk the mascarpone, sugar, and vanilla extract in a bowl with a hand mixer until smooth.
- Add in the chocolate mixture.
- Spoon the mixture into silicone muffin tins and freeze for 4 hours.

Sweet Honey Panna Cotta

6 Servings

Preparation Time: 10 min + cooling time

Ingredients

- 3 tbsps honey
- 1½ tsps vanilla extract
- 1 cup chocolate chips, melted
- 3½ gelatin leaves
- 1½ cups heavy cream
- 3 cups milk

Directions

- Put the gelatin leaves in a bowl and cover it with cold water.
- Leave to soak for about 5 minutes.
- Put a pan over medium heat and add in heavy cream, milk, honey, and vanilla; stir it and bring it to a boil.
- When it boils, remove it from the heat, then strain the gelatin and fold it in the cream mixture, stir until the gelatin has dissolved.
- Transfer it in the 4 cups and let cool at room temperature, then put in the fridge for 2 hours.

- When cooled, dip the cups in hot water and put them onto serving plates.
- Serve with melted chocolate.

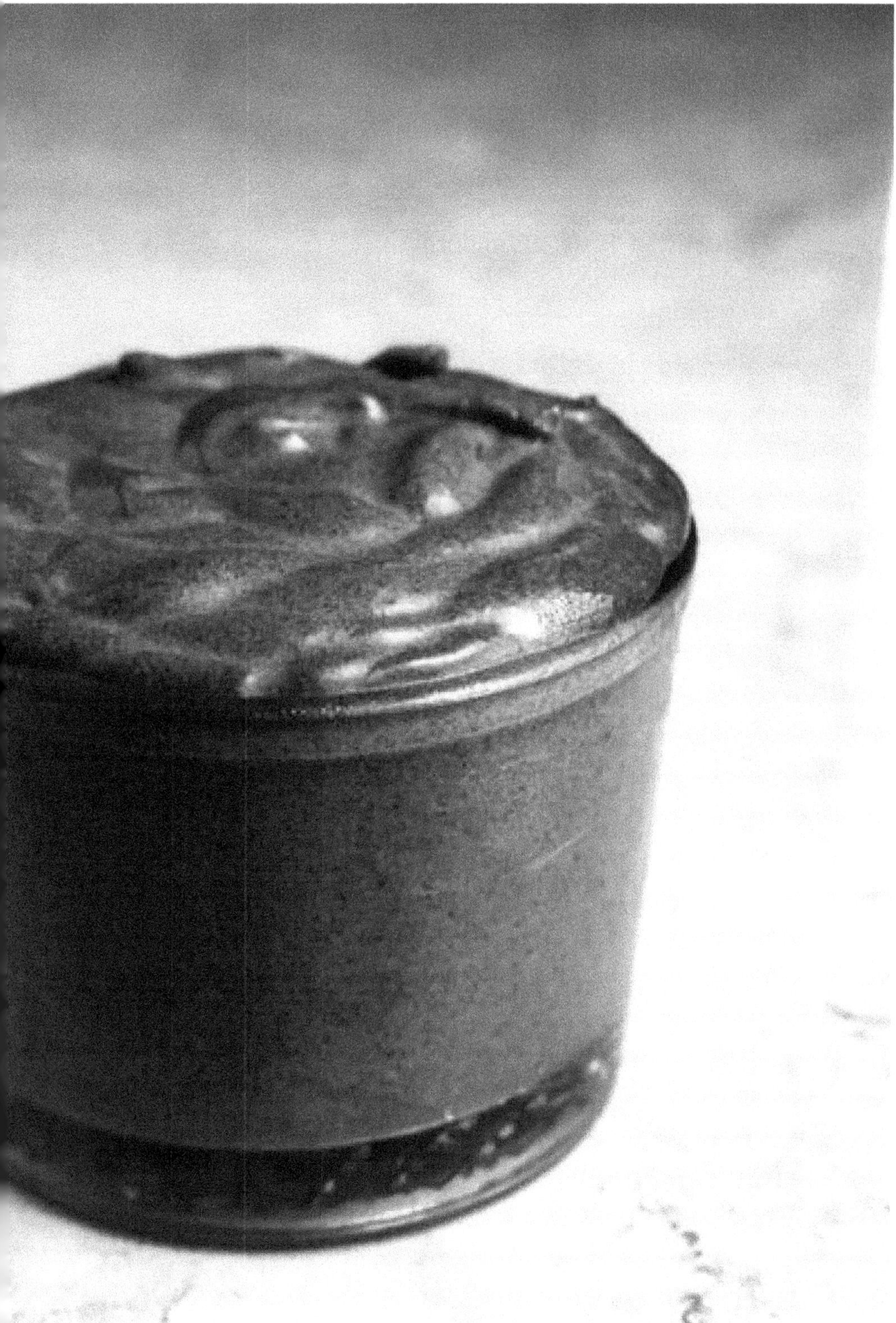

Caramel with Whipped Cream

7 Servings

Preparation Time: 10 minutes

Ingredients

- 1½ tbsps vanilla extract
- 1 cup of sugar for custard
- 2½ cups heavy whipping cream
- 1½ egg yolk
- 7 eggs
- 2½ cups milk
- 1 cup sugar for caramel

Directions

- Make the caramel: warm the sugar for the caramel in a deep pan.
- Add 2-3 tbsps of water, and bring to a boil.
- Cook until the caramel turns golden brown, then reduce the heat.
- Divide the caramel between 5 metal tins. Let it cool.
- Preheat the oven to 345ºF.
- Mix the eggs, egg yolk, remaining sugar, lemon zest, and vanilla extract in a bowl.

115

- Add the milk in it and beat again until well combined.
- Transfer the mixture into each caramel-lined pot and put them into a deep baking tin.
- Fill over with the remaining hot water.
- Bake for about 45-50 minutes. Using tongs take out the pot and let them cool for at least 4 hours in the fridge.
- Transfer onto a dish. Serve with dollops of whipped cream.

Chocolate and Hazelnut Chocolate Bars
14 Servings

Preparation Time: 1 hr 15 minutes

Ingredients

- 1 tsp salt
- 6 ounces dark chocolate
- 1 cup hazelnut butter
- 1 cup toasted hazelnuts, chopped
- 4 tbsps sugar

Directions

- Microwave the hazelnut butter and chocolate for about 90 seconds.
- Remove and add in the sugar. Spread the chocolate evenly on a line of cookie sheets with waxed paper.
- On the top, scatter the hazelnuts and sprinkle some salt.
- Refrigerate it for about one hour.

Chocolate Pudding in a Cup

4 Servings

Preparation Time: 10 minutes

Ingredients

- 4½ oz milk
- 6 tbsps olive oil
- 1 tsp baking powder
- Whipped cream for topping
- 4 eggs
- 4½ oz flour
- 12 tbsps sugar
- 12 tbsps cocoa powder

Directions

- Mix the flour, sugar, cocoa powder, espresso powder, eggs, milk, olive oil, and baking powder in a bowl.
- Put the mix into mugs ¾ way up and cook in a microwave for about 70 seconds.
- Remove it from the microwave and churn the whipping cream on the cakes and serve.

Hazelnut with Berry Truffles

10 Servings

Preparation Time: 6 min + cooling time

Ingredients

- 1 cup berry preserves
- 2 tbsps sugar
- 2 tbsps olive oil
- 7 oz chocolate chips
- 1½ cup raw hazelnuts
- 1½ tbsp flaxseeds

Directions

- In a blender, blend the hazelnuts and flax seeds for about 45 seconds until smoothly crushed; add the berry preserves and 2 tbsps of sugar in it.
- Blend further for almost 1 minute until well combined.
- Make 1-inch balls of the mixture, put on a parchment paper-lined baking sheet, and freeze it for about 1 hour.
- In a microwave, melt the chocolate chips, oil, and 1tbsp of sugar for about 90 seconds.
- Stir the truffles to coat in the chocolate mixture, put it on the baking sheet, and freeze further for at least 2 hours.

Chocolate Mousse with Strawberries

6 Servings

Preparation Time: 30 minutes

Ingredients

- 1½ cups of fresh strawberries, sliced
- 1 ½vanilla extract
- 1½ tbsps. of sugar
- 4 eggs
- 1 tsp salt
- 12 oz dark chocolate, melted
- 1½ cup heavy cream

Directions

- Whip the cream in a medium mixing bowl until very soft.
- Add the eggs, vanilla extract, and sugar in it; whisk to combine the mixture. Then Fold into the chocolate.
- Transfer the mousse between glasses, top with the strawberry slices, and chill in the fridge for at least 30 minutes before serving.

SOUPS

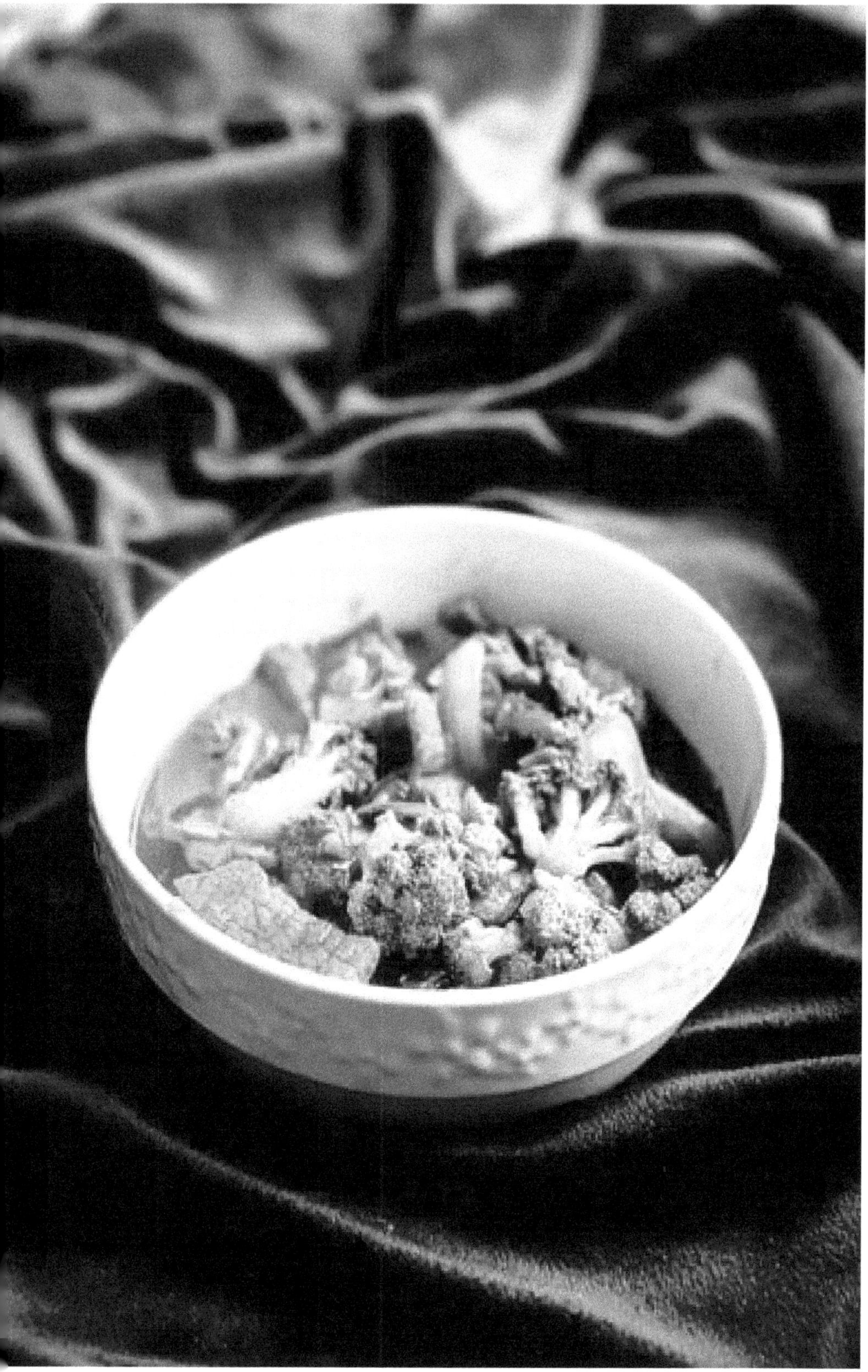

Classical Egg Drop Soup

4 Servings

Preparation Time: 15 minutes

Ingredients

- 1 tbsp cornstarch
- 1 tbsp dried minced onion
- 1 tbsp dried parsley
- 2 eggs
- 2 cubes chicken bouillon
- 6 cups water
- 1 cup chopped up carrots
- ½ cup finely shredded cabbage

Directions

- Combine water, bouillon, parsley, cabbage, carrots, and onion flakes in a saucepan, and then bring to a boil.
- Beat the eggs lightly and mix them into the soup.
- Dissolve cornstarch with a little water.
- Mix until smooth and mix into the soup.
- Let it boil until the soup thickens.

Yummy Hot and Sour Soup

4 Servings

Preparation Time: 25 minutes

Ingredients

- ½ tbsp sesame oil
- 1 cup fresh bean sprouts
- 1 egg, lightly beaten
- 1 tbsp black pepper
- 1 tbsp ground ginger
- 3 tbsps white vinegar
- 3 tbsps soy sauce
- ¼ pound. Sliced mushrooms
- ½ pound. Tofu chopped up
- 2 tbsps corn starch
- 3 ½ cups chicken broth

Directions

- Mix corn starch and ¼ cup chicken broth and put aside.
- Over high-level heat, place a pan, then combine and boil: pepper, ginger, vinegar, soy sauce, mushrooms, tofu, and chicken broth.

- Once boiling, add the corn starch mixture. Mix constantly and reduce the fire. Once the concoction is thickened, drop the slightly beaten egg while mixing vigorously.
- Add bean sprouts and for one to two minutes, let simmering.
- Remove from fire and pour to serving bowls and enjoy while hot.

Green Vegan Soup

6 Servings

Preparation Time: 20 minutes

Ingredients

- 1 medium head cauliflower cut into bite-sized florets
- 1 medium white onion peeled and diced
- 2 cloves garlic peeled and diced
- 1 bay leaf crushed
- 5-ounce watercress
- Fresh spinach
- 1-liter vegetable stock or bone broth
- 1 cup cream or coconut milk + 6 tbsp for garnish
- Quarter cup ghee or coconut oil
- 1 tbsp salt or to taste
- Freshly ground black pepper
- Fresh herbs such as parsley or chives for garnish

Directions

- Set the fire on a medium-high level, place a Dutch oven greased with ghee. Once hot, sauté garlic for a minute.

- Add onions and sauté until soft and translucent, about 5 minutes.
- Add cauliflower florets and crushed bay leaf. Mix well and cook for 5 minutes.
- Mix in watercress and spinach. Sauté for 3 minutes.
- Add vegetable stock and bring to a boil.
- When cauliflower is crisp-tender, mix in coconut milk.
- Season with pepper and salt.
- With a hand blender, puree soup until smooth and creamy. Serve and enjoy.

Cauliflower Masala Soup

4 Servings

Preparation Time: 35 minutes

Ingredients

- 1 tbsp salt
- 1 tbsp ground turmeric
- 1 tbsp ground coriander
- 2 tbsps cumin seeds
- 1 tbsp dark mustard seeds.
- 1 cup water
- cups beef broth
- 1 head cauliflower chopped up
- 3 carrots chopped up
- 1 large onion chopped up
- 2 tbsps coconut oil
- Chopped up cilantro for topping
- Crushed red pepper to taste
- Black pepper to taste
- 1 tbsp lemon juice

Directions

- On medium high-level fire, place a large, heavy-bottomed pan and heat coconut oil.
- Once hot, sauté garlic cloves for a minute.

- Add carrots and continue sautéing for 4 minutes more.
- Add turmeric, coriander, cumin, mustard seeds, and cauliflower.
- Sauté for 5 minutes.
- Add water and beef broth and simmer for 10 to 15 minutes.
- Turn off the fire and pour to the blender.
- Puree until smooth and creamy.
- Return to pan, continue simmering for another ten minutes.
- Season with crushed red pepper, lemon juice, pepper, and salt.
- To serve, garnish with cilantro, and enjoy.

Spiced Ginger Carrot Soup

6 Servings

Preparation Time: 40 minutes

Ingredients

- ¼ cup Greek yogurt
- 2 tbsps fresh lime juice
- 5 cups low-salt chicken broth
- 1 ½ tbsp finely grated lime peel
- 2 cups of carrots, peeled, finely sliced into rounds
- 2 cups chopped up onions
- 1 tbsp minced and peeled fresh ginger
- ½ tbsp curry powder
- Tbsp expeller-pressed sunflower oil
- ½ tbsp yellow mustard seeds.
- 1 tbsp coriander seeds

Directions

- In a food processor, grind mustard seeds and coriander into a powder.
- On medium high-level fire, place a large pan and heat oil.
- Add curry powder and powdered seeds and sauté for a minute.

- Add ginger, cook for a minute.
- Add lime peel, carrots, and onions.
- Sauté for 3 minutes or until onions are softened.
- Season with pepper and salt.
- Add broth and bring to a boil.
- Reduce fire to a simmer and simmer uncovered for 30 minutes or until carrots are tender.
- Cool broth slightly and puree in batches. Return pureed carrots into the pan.
- Add lime juice, add more pepper and salt to taste.
- Pour to a serving bowl, drizzle with yogurt, and serve.

Zoodles with Ginger Egg Drop Soup

4 Servings

Preparation Time: 15 minutes

Ingredients

- ½ tsp red pepper flakes
- 2 cups finely sliced scallions, divided
- 2 cups, plus 1 tbsp water, divided
- 2 tbsps extra virgin olive oil
- 2 tbsps minced ginger
- 2 tbsps corn starch
- 2 large eggs, beaten
- Medium to large zucchini, spiralized into noodles
- 2 cups shiitake mushrooms, sliced
- 5 tbsps low-sodium tamari sauce or soy sauce
- 5 cups vegetable broth, divided
- Salt & pepper to taste

Directions

- Set the fire on a medium-high level, place a large pan and add oil.
- Once the oil is hot, mix in ginger and sauté for two minutes.
- Mix in a tbsp of water and shiitake mushrooms.

- Cook for 5 minutes or until mushrooms starts to give off liquid.
- Mix in 1 ½ cups scallions, tamari sauce, red pepper flakes, remaining water, and 7 cups of vegetable broth.
- Mix well and bring to a boil.
- In the meantime, in a small bowl, whisk well cornstarch and the remaining cup of vegetable broth and set aside.
- Once the pan is boiling, slowly pour in eggs while mixing the pan continuously.
- Mix well.
- Add the cornstarch slurry into the pan and mix well. Continue mixing every now and then until thickened, about 5 minutes.
- Taste and adjust seasoning with pepper and salt.
- Mix in zoodles and cook until heated for about 2 minutes.
- Serve with a sprinkle of remaining scallions and enjoy.

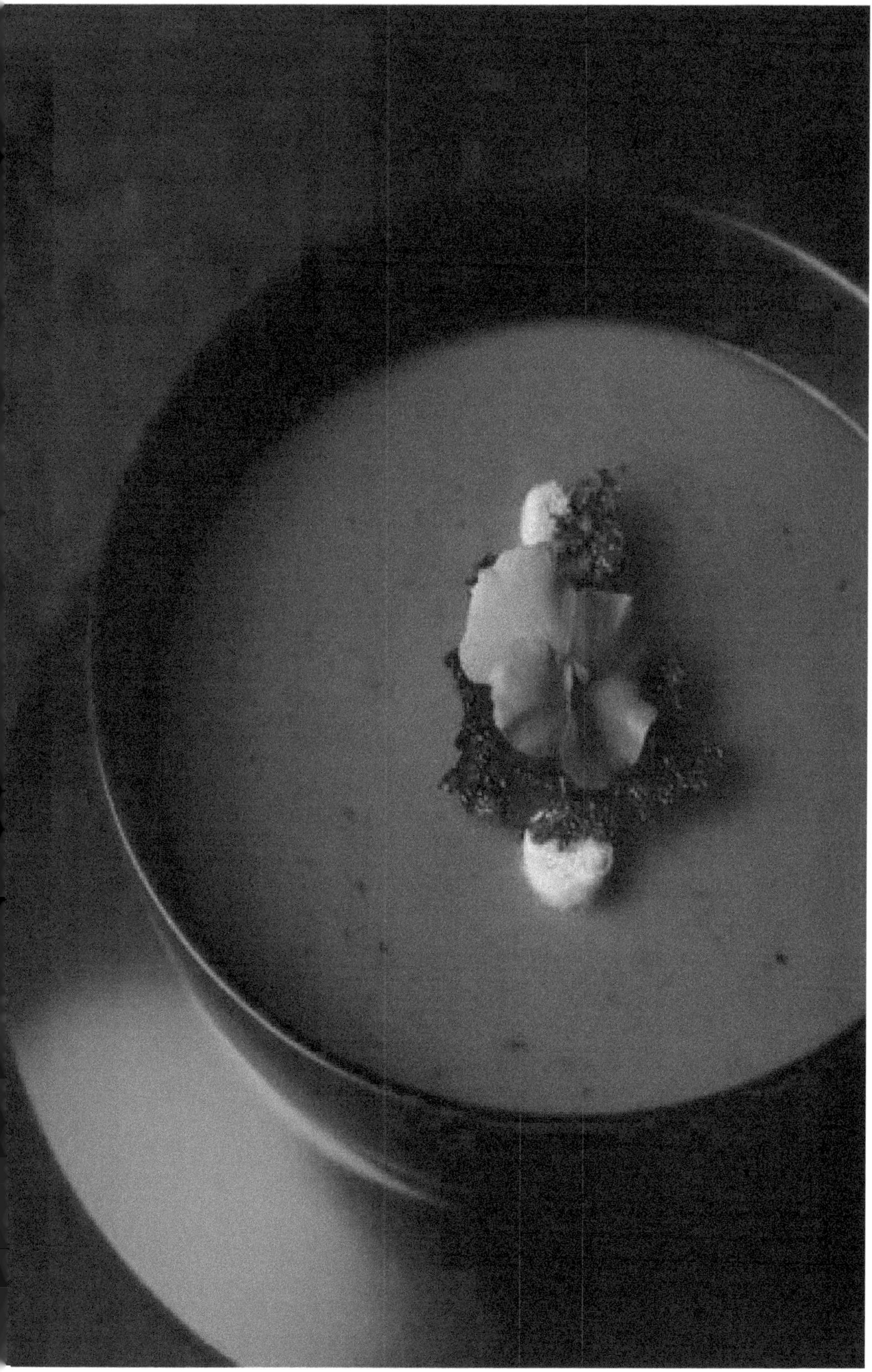

Corn with Cream Soup

4 Servings

Preparation Time: 20 minutes

Ingredients

- 4 slices crisp-cooked bacon, crushed
- 2 tbsps cornstarch
- Quarter cup water
- 2 tbsps soy sauce
- 4 cups chicken broth
- 1 (14.75 ounce) can cream-style corn
- 2 egg whites
- Quarter tbsp salt
- 1 tbsp sherry
- Half pound. Skinless, boneless chicken breast meat finely chopped up

Directions

- Combine chicken with the sherry, egg whites, salt in a bowl.
- Mix in the cream-style corn.
- Mix well.
- Boil the soy sauce and chicken broth in a wok. Then mix in the chicken mixture while continue boiling.

- Then simmer for about 3 minutes, frequently mix to avoid burning.
- Mix corn starch and water until well combined. Mix to the simmering broth while constantly mixing until it slightly thickens.
- Cook for about 2 minutes more.
- Serve tpped with the crushed bacon.

Lightning Source UK Ltd.
Milton Keynes UK
UKHW021024240621
386074UK00004B/51